PRAISES FOR MAKE PEACE WITH FAT

"When reading Mihaela's book and absorbing all the insightful, practical and well-researched information she presents, one sentence immediately stands out to me: "Once you understand WHY, the HOW becomes 10X easier." Mihaela seems to make this her mantra throughout her book. She doesn't just share why certain dietary and lifestyle changes make sense but also presents the scientific rationale behind her explanations. In many instances, she illustrates biochemical processes, hormonal interactions or complex intricacies of the human body with visual, easy-to-follow graphs or diagrams. This and also the fact that almost half her book is all about taking action and implementing new knowledge makes this an information-packed but very approachable read for both practitioners and anybody seeking to take their health into their own hands.

When talking about her diet and lifestyle during her childhood and adolescence in Communist Romania, Mihaela remembers that it was "simple, easy, healing" due to the absence of distractions like processed foods, TV and other comforts. She takes the reader on a journey how she grew up, how much community was valued and also how physically tough people were. Not only does she share some insights into how life used to be for her and her family, but also the health challenges she faced later on and how she struggled for years to get a handle on those.
We are blessed that Mihaela has decided to put her story, her vast knowledge and experience to paper and I have no doubt that she will inspire many people to follow in her footsteps. To explore dietary and lifestyle options, learn about their body and take action towards improved and long-lasting vitality."

— **Patricia Daly**, Nutritional Therapist, Co-Author of "The Ketogenic Kitchen", www.patriciadaly.com

"I thought I knew a lot about nutrition, but this fantastic book taught me so much more. Mihaela takes the mystery out of personalizing a healthy high-fat, low-carbohydrate diet and explains the benefits of fasting. I highly recommend this book, which is now my go-to resource for healthy eating."

—**Keith Holden, MD**, Author of Power of the Mind in Health and Healing

"In an easy to follow, conversational style, Mihaela makes the act of eating to support good health that has become complex and almost foreign in our present food environment, simple and attainable. Her book not only teaches the science behind the innate wisdom of our bodies, but takes us, step by step, through a journey of transformation towards optimal health."

—**Maria E. Pizano-Balatovis, MS, RD, CDE**, Public Health Nutritionist

"This book can make many of your health and life dreams come true. It gives you a deep insight into how food can heal your body. It makes you aware of the many health benefits associated with following a low-carbohydrate, high-fat diet and most importantly, this book gives you practical advice, the "how to," from cleaning up your pantry and refrigerator and restocking them with high-fat, low-carb whole foods, to kitchen equipment and cooking healthy and innovative recipes, it covers them all. Nothing is left for guessing or "googling". I'm confident that Make Peace with Fat will build up your nutrition knowledge and it will help you become clear and laser-focused on what you need to do to take charge of your health, as it helped me."

—**L. Vasile**, Teacher of English and International School Project Coordinator

"Once you accept the power of food, you need a guide for how to use it. Make Peace With Fat is that instruction manual. With easy-to-follow, scientific explanations, step-by-step instructions, detailed food list, a low-carb, high-fat whole foods menu, recipes and loads of resources, anyone can learn to eat their way toward better health."

—**Lauren Griffin**, Chief Operating Officer, Griffin Concierge Medical

"Everyone can benefit from reading this book and implementing Dr. Telecan's practices. Whether you are trying to lose weight, overcome a chronic disease or improve your health for longevity, this book will show you the way. I have followed this advice and reaped the rewards of healing and exceptional health. Purchasing this book will be an investment in your future health."

—**Pat Janco**, Dog Mamma and Healing With Foods client

"A Must Read! This book is a must read for everyone since Dr. Telecan is passionate about helping people get past the fads and conflicting or confusing information regarding wellness and nutrition to provide a clear, simple method to how to think about food to improve its impact on our overall health first and foremost, but to benefit from the secondary outcomes we all want – to feel better, to lose fat and maintain a healthy weight, to increase energy and gain clarity and focus – all through a lifestyle that is simple and effective to follow. I selected Dr. Telecan to be my nutritionist and wellness practitioner for her in-depth medical knowledge and because her methodology is based on sharing the "why". Rather than giving me menus to follow, Mihaela armed me with the information I needed to make good decisions that I could live with long term. After working with Dr. Telecan for three months, I developed healthy habits, am back to wearing skinny jeans again (without the bulge flowing over the top) and I have eliminated medications that I had been dependent on for years. I highly recommend this book to anyone who wants to gain the knowledge required to truly live a healthier, stronger and more confident life."

—**Jeannette Kraar, CEO**, Performance Management International LLC and Healing With Foods client

"Doctors have been at war with fat for decades. We are slowly seeing the light. "Make Peace with Fat" is the nutrition course we never had in medical school. A must-read for any practitioner looking for the nutritional tools to help their patients heal."

—**Radley Griffin, MD**, Founder, Griffin Concierge Medical

"We need to thank Mihaela Telecan for writing this book! She gave a good explanation of how the human body works and how our food affects it. Her personal story gives this book a genuine touch – this is honest information coming from the heart. I warmly recommend it!"

—**Dr Natasha Campbell-McBride, MD**, creator of the GAPS Nutritional Protocol and author of several books on health.

Thank you Mihaela Telecan for writing such a concise and comprehensive explanation of how food affects the body. A great read I wish I had had it in my university days. A must read for students of various health fields. I highly recommend it to all health practitioners and for everyone who wishes to improve health. The statement: 'Let food be thy medicine and thy medicine be thy food' takes on a more practical dimension with the explanations of the why and how.

—**Dr. Olivia Kojman, DVM., DOM., AP.**

"There is much confusion these days about what to eat. If you take the time to learn how food affects your health, you'll be compelled to eat well. This book offers you that experience."

—**Beth Zupec-Kania, RDN, CD**

"In *Make Peace with Fat*, Mihaela Telecan provides a convincing rationale for following a low-carb, high-fat diet based on whole, unprocessed foods. After recounting her compelling personal journey to wellness, she shares evidence-based information about the benefits of this way of eating for digestive health, hormonal regulation, and weight loss, along with easily understood tips and guidance for making this a permanent lifestyle change. As a fellow registered dietitian and certified diabetes educator, I wholeheartedly recommend this book for nutrition professionals and doctors, as well as anyone interested in achieving optimal health with a real food approach."

—**Franziska Spritzler, RD, CDE**, *The Low Carb Dietiitan's Guide to Health and Beauty*

"In Make Peace with Fat, Mihaela reinforces the notion that foods in their whole and unprocessed forms—which includes nourishing animal foods and animal fats—is optimal for the human body. If you're struggling with chronic illness or metabolic disease, you'll be both informed and empowered to take back your health with real food."

—**Lily Nichols, RD, CDE**, Bestselling author of Real Food for Gestational Diabetes

"Wow! Mihaela Telecan has taken the science of both metabolic disease as well as many of the autoimmune issues facing so many today and makes this simple, clear, and comprehensible. More importantly she outlines the steps to reset and restore health using real food. As a Family Physician we must teach these approaches to the next generation of health care workers who will spend their careers dealing with chronic disease, not acute illness and injury."

— **Mark Cucuzzella, MD** FAAFP Professor West Virginia University School of Medicine *WVU Center for Diabetes and Metabolic Health*

"In "Make Peace With Fat", Mihaela Telecan takes the reader through her own gut and health-healing journey, stopping along the way to explain in relatable language what she learned through her many years of study. Her passion for helping others is evident on every page as she skillfully guides readers through the first few critical steps needed to get on the path to better health. What an incredible resource for the growing low-carb community!"-

— **Miriam Kalamian, EdM, MS, CNS**. Author of Keto for Cancer: Ketogenic Metabolic Therapy as a Targeted Nutritional Strategy (Chelsea Green Publishing; 2017)

MAKE PEACE WITH FAT is written by Dr. Mihaela Telecan, a graduate of the Institute for Integrative Nutrition, where they completed a cutting edge curriculum in nutrition and health coaching taught by the world's leading experts in health and wellness. I recommend you read this book and be in touch with Dr. Telecan to see how she can help you successfully achieve your goals.

— **Joshua Rosenthal, MScEd**, Founder/Director, Institute for Integrative Nutrition

Transform Your Mind, Body and Health

MAKE PEACE WITH FAT

Transform Your Mind, Body and Health

MAKE PEACE WITH FAT

Applying ancestral wisdom and modern nutrition
to reverse metabolic diseases, reset hunger, increase energy
and maximize performance

Mihaela A. Telecan, DVM, RD

ISBN-13: 978-1979139564
ISBN-10: 1979139563
LCCN: 2017917564

Book editing by Dr. Susan Moore, MD.
Cover and interior design by PrintDesigner.ro
Author photography by Janet Chrisakis

DEDICATION

I dedicate this book, to my son, Andrei, my husband, Luiz, and to my parents, Dumitru and Elena. Without your unconditional love, support, and continuous encouragement this book would not have been written. I'm forever grateful for being your mom, your wife, and your daughter. Thank you!

CONTENT

INTRODUCTION

Food and eating have become more and more complicated over time. It used to be that we knew what to eat, how much to eat and when to eat. Somehow, we knew when we were full. We didn't have to journal it, or to log our macro and micronutrients in a fancy app to know if we were doing the right thing. Eating was a very natural process, just like breathing. We don't have to think how many breaths we should be taking in a day, minute or hour; how deep a breath should be when we are running versus sitting; or if we are breathing the "correct air composition"—perhaps we need a bit more oxygen and less nitrogen. Breathing comes very naturally; we don't have to overthink it.

However, when it comes to food and what we eat, it got complicated, to the point that we now have nutritionists, doctors, trainers, chiropractors, and even the government telling us what we should eat, how often and how much.

It's paradoxical that I'm saying this, because I'm a nutritionist writing this book about what to eat, how much to eat and how often to eat.

You, me and every other human on this planet instinctively know when to eat and how much to eat. But, somehow, we forgot how to do it. From a very young age we were forced to ignore our own intuition, our body's wisdom.

Does this sound familiar to you?

> *"Eat everything on your plate."*
> *"But I'm full mommy."*
> *"No, you have to eat it all."*
> *"Come eat, is lunch time."*
> *"I'm not hungry yet."*
> *"It doesn't matter, it's time to eat."*

For most of us that's what happened growing up: we were told to eat and we had to eat, even when we were not hungry or when our body didn't send us any signals indicating the need to eat. Over time, we learned to override the body's queues for hunger, thirst, and satiety and followed external commands, such as those coming from our parents, teachers, doctors, etc.

Not only have we lost the inner wisdom, but the wisdom that was passed on from generation to generation: traditional wisdom. The "experts," the government and, worst of all, the food industry took over and are telling us what to eat, how often and how much.

So, here I am, a "nutrition expert," writing a book about how to eat and how to use food as medicine. Why would I do that when I believe we each have our own guiding system within us? When there are so many health, nutrition and diet books already? Well, I happen to see things from a slightly different perspective. I'm writing this book, not to give you another scientific fact nor to make you more confused and overwhelmed, but to raise your awareness about the immense power you have to heal. I want to empower you; to give you permission to listen to your inner wisdom; to invite you to stop and question what you're told by the "experts," and to look back and learn from traditional and ancestral wisdom. My goal is to also to give you the practical tools you need to take action.

Back in 2012, when I started my private coaching practice, I made the following public statement as my commitment:

"My commitment to you is to raise your awareness about the power that lies within you; educate you and help transform your health and life by using the limitless power of real whole foods, movement, nature and ancient wisdom. Through your transformation we will change the health and happiness of the world one woman at a time."

I remained faithful to this! It is still my mission and my purpose in life to help transform millions of lives, one life at a time.

Awareness-Empowerment-Action!

Mihaela A. Telecan

HOW DID IT START?

I was born in a "different time and a different era" in Communist Romania. I lived my first 17 years of life under Communism. What does this have to do with food and lifestyle? I say everything!

When I moved to the United States, I felt like I was an alien, like I was literally coming from another planet. I craved walking and bumping into people more than anything else. I longed for public transportation. I felt overwhelmed when I walked for the first time into a supermarket with all the bright aisles, and multitudes of packaged foods and perfect looking vegetables that had no taste. I was longing for a tomato that actually tasted like one and milk that had fat floating on top so that I could, just like back home, turn it into yogurt. Life in the USA was very different than life was back in Romania.

I said to myself, *"Is this an experimental life? Is somebody trying to see how the human race will turn out if they have all the comfort one can possibly imagine, if they have easy access to food, if they don't even have to walk because everything is convenient and comfortable, from drive-thrus to escalators, dish washers, and microwave ovens?"*

I went through a huge learning curve to adapt to my new environment, from language to food and movement. I can say that I managed to learn, adapt and, ultimately, thrive in my new environment. And you can, too. You can learn, adapt and change as you choose to.

For you, it may not be new as in a new country, but it may be a new way of living. It may not involve learning a new language, though some of the terms in this book may be new. For you, it may mean learning to drop some of the modern day comfort and walk more, cook more (from scratch, not using the microwave), shopping from the local farmer's market foods that don't have a food label or a portion size assigned to them. It may be learning to trust your intuition. You may need to learn to feel when you are full and satisfied, to eat only when you are hungry, and, when you are upset, to cry and call a friend to talk about it, instead of reaching for the ice cream.

Don't get me wrong, I love my life here in the USA. In fact, when I'm writing this book, I have 17 years of life experience in the USA and I would not want to live anywhere else.

Now, I'd like to take you back in time, to my childhood days, so you can better understand why I felt like I was from another planet, from "a different time and era," when I first moved to the states.

Just to put things into perspective, growing up in Communist Romania meant basically that there were no food advertisements, no vending machines, no soft drinks, no processed foods and no school lunch programs dictated by the government or by big food industries. It meant that we ate what we cultivated in our garden and the animal products from the animals we were raising. We ate what my mother or grandmother prepared from scratch, using fresh whole food ingredients that were locally and seasonally available.

I remember very vividly being 18 years old—it was soon after communism was abolished—when, for the first time, I tasted Coca-Cola. Can you guess my re-action to this beverage? I spit it out! I said to myself, *"This is not for human consumption."* I guess not having access to processed foods and having sugar from homemade desserts usually once a week was a blessing in disguise, as my taste buds did not get "corrupted" and acquainted with the addictive flavors of processed foods.

This may not be your case at all, as you may have been exposed to processed foods that are high in sugar and vegetable oils, along with processed beverages, such as Coca-Cola or Pepsi, from a very young age, and that perhaps did not serve you well. But do not worry! You can retrain your taste buds to recognize the delicious flavors of real fresh whole foods and to actually love them.

Growing up, I could see my parents and grandparents, my whole family, working together. We lived a simple, yet hard life that was less convenient and less comfortable than the life we know here in the States. We worked the land together. We cooked together. We chopped wood for the winter and we also played together a lot. We hardly had any TV time and no computers at all, as those were the days when communism didn't allow access to information from the Western World. They kept us "trapped in there."

It wasn't good, but it wasn't all bad either. What could have been good in that you may ask?

It allowed us to spend more time with each other, to strengthen our familial and social ties. We had plenty of time to play and to read books. We didn't have more hours in a day back then than we have now, but it seemed like we did.

Often, I hear my clients saying, or I find myself thinking, *"I don't have enough time."* Then I look at how I spend my time. How much time do I spend in front of the screen (TV, computer, smartphone, Facebook)? Is it true that we don't have time for what's truly important to us? Or that we don't make the time? We allow "time thieves" into our lives and we lose awareness of it. We fool ourselves into believing that we don't have time to shop, to cook, to walk, to meet with friends or family. I'm sure you know what I mean.

I remember using the petroleum lamp on the nights electricity was cut off, and playing games or telling stories. Rationed electricity created room for family time. Having rationed gasoline made it so that we didn't travel very much and we hung out locally with our friends and family. Food was also rationed.

When I moved to the city to attend high school, I had to buy bread and sometimes milk from the store. There were always long lines to get those foods. Sometimes, I would stand in line for hours and the food would run out right when it was my turn to get my portion. Then, I would go to another store hoping to find it there. If I was lucky to get there and to still find bread or milk, I had to show my card to be marked off that I received my ration for the day. I know this was the wrong way to operate, but, sometimes, I feel like that's what we need today in Western countries: food rations, not gastric bypass surgery.

It seems so foreign to live that way, but that's how I grew up. I guess that's why if you ask me today to stand in line to take a ride in an amusement park I would say to you, *"There is no way you are gonna see me standing in line for anything after the amount of time I spent in lines for food!"* I think I developed "line phobia."

I believe that, because we didn't have the influence from the food industry, we based our food consumption solely on traditional wisdom, which had been passed on from generation to generation. Growing up, I learned from my mother how to make food from scratch; food that included—believe it or not—the skin and the fat of the animal, along with their organs, even the brain. When an animal was killed, whether it was chicken, cow, lamb or pig, every part of that animal was consumed. I could see my mother cleaning the stomach and the intestines of the pig to be used to make sausages and a traditional Romanian dish called "toba," which was made out of some of the skin, ears, tongue and other organs of the pig with lots of gelatin extracted from cooking the pig feet.

Since refrigeration as a storage method was either not possible or very limited, we preserved vegetables through fermentation and home canning, both of fruits and vegetables. In the summer we made fruit preserves for the winter and every fall we filled up the cellars with jars of ferments and preserves. From sauerkraut to tomato sauce, we made them all. We also made our own cheese, yogurt, sourdough bread and even noodles for chicken noodle soup.

This made my definition of food, and my perception of what it takes to acquire food and to turn it into "meals," very different than that of most people living in industrialized countries who are accustomed to getting prepackaged foods that they just stick into the microwave or pick up at the drive-thru.

And, there's more to it.

Aside from food, other aspects of that lifestyle were very different as well. We felt the cold in the winter while walking to school, waiting for busses or trains. That's not to say that our home didn't have centralized heating. We had a furnace in each room. We made a wood fire in the furnace, during the day when we were home. At night if we slept too deep and nobody woke up to add more wood to the fire, we woke up in the morning in a freezing cold room.

The opposite happened in the summer. We were extremely hot, because we didn't have air conditioned homes, cars or buses. I remember getting nosebleeds in the summer, because of the heat.

We performed a lot of physical labor to work the land for food. In the summer, the men cut the grass manually and, then, when it was dry, we collected the hay, also manually. We worked in the garden every day, plugging weeds and doing more intense tasks when it was harvest time. It was so much physical and manual labor to grow the food we ate that it made me not want to ever grow my own food again.

Now, of course, I feel differently about this. At the time, in my teen years, it acted as a motivating factor and it made me study hard so I would have a profession that would pay me well, to afford to buy the food from the farmers. I'm very grateful my parents supported me in every way they could, so I was able to fulfil my professional dream.

I hope that sharing a snippet of my early upbringing, what life was like in "another era," helps you to better understand why my definition of life-style in general, and that of food in particular, is fundamentally different than that of most people, including health professionals that were raised in societies that offered comfort and convenience, both in lifestyle as well as in food. I believe that I'm able to pull out the best from the two cultures which I was blessed to live in, add to it a good dose of science, and create a unique recipe for health, healing and happiness.

"Simple, Easy, Healing!" In fact, the unique upbringing, my own healing journey, true passion and many years of studies made possible for this book to come to life. You are probably asking what my health challenges were and what studies helped me come to this point, where I'm sitting down and writing a book. A book which I hope it's worth reading and it will help you transform your health and life.

I didn't start with my professional journey as a nutritionist or dietitian. No, even my professional journey was a fifteen-year-long journey. I'm glad I didn't give up. I persevered and I persued my dreams, and now, I live my purpose - helping individuals transform their health and life through food and lifestyle. In fact, my healing journey and professional journey went in parallel. My sickness and my desire to heal with food are what gave me the courage to say no to what was considered a profitable career and follow my true passion for health and healing.

When I turned 18, I was admitted to veterinary school. I had to pass a very difficult exam to get in and then I spent the next six years studying to become a veterinarian. I loved the science and learning about animals health and healing, but I wasn't passionate about it. It was a good paying job, but my heart wasn't in it. I always had a natural inclination for health and performance. I was passionate about alternative ways to heal the body, and I was interested in learning how to optimize physical performance and to prevent premature aging.

Growing up, I was blessed with good health. I strongly believe that the simple life with good food and close proximity with nature, family and friends was a big contributing factor. However, in my 20s, while in veterinary school, I realized that I had major constipation. That's when I began to pay attention to my body. I slowed down a bit and paid attention to how I felt and how food was affecting me.

It took me twenty years to figure out how to heal with foods. I'm glad I persevered on my healing journey and didn't give up. I'm in a far better place now than I was twenty-five years ago.

On my healing journey, I traveled the road of high fiber diet with loads of wheat bran and psyllium husk. I took the paths of raw vegan, "cooked" vegan, and vegetarian (lacto-ovo) diets.

Like every person out there that's trying to heal with foods, I thought the answer to my constipation was a high fiber plant-based diet. Especially for constipation, having more fiber had to be a good thing, right?

It's worth mentioning that I had a bunch of tests done to figure out why I only had a bowel movement once every 7 to 10 days. I went to the local gastroenterology clinic, and I requested to be admitted into the hospital to figure out why I was constipated.

For the first time in 20 years of life, I was hospitalized.

I wanted to know what was going on inside my gut. Why? Well, I got scared to death when I learned in my veterinary studies about the health dangers of chronic constipation (one being cancer). I wasn't feeling bad yet, but I didn't want to wait to feel bad before I took action.

That's why I'm a big believer in awareness. How can you change if you don't even know you need to change? You don't know what you don't know. It's another way of saying, ignorance stops progress. Knowledge is power, especially if you use it to take action. Actions lead to results.

So, I was given the diagnosis of mega-colon (mega=large, colon=large intestine). The doctors told me some people are born with a big nose, I was born with a big colon, and they could fix it for me with surgery. They could cut me open, make my colon smaller and my bowel function would normalize. As you can probably guess, that didn't sit well with a young, slender, athletic girl, let alone with one that wanted to do everything naturally.

Since it was about the gut, common sense was screaming at me that *food must be the solution*. So, my healing with food quest began.

For the first ten years of my healing journey, I tried to increase fiber and water. I slowly removed animal protein from my diet and, when I turned 30, I was a hopeful raw vegan. I really thought I found the solution to my now uncomfortable, not-responsive-to-diet constipation. I was determined not to take laxatives, as I knew how damaging to the liver those were. Plus, they cause dependence and then I would have a bigger problem to deal with. Instead, I was getting my bowels to move with Senna tea and herbs such as Cascara Sagrada.

The raw diet didn't make a dent and colonics were not the solution either. Daily enemas became my management. I knew that I had to have at a minimum one bowel movement per day. So, for years and years (I lost count of how many), I did a daily enema. Don't ask me how those days were. All I choose to remember is it was worth doing every single one of them to prevent colon cancer, liver toxicity from drugs, or dependency induced by drugs or herbs.

But there had to be another way, a better way.

For the next 10 years, I continued my journey from raw vegan to lacto-ovo vegetarian, but not only did my constipation never resolve, my overall health began to deteriorate. It was subtle. I began to feel cold all the time (imagine living in Miami and feeling cold—not good, right?). My skin turned yellow, glands in my neck were swollen all the time, and the doctors were telling me that must be normal for me.

I didn't like that answer.

There had to be a reason for why they were swollen. Years later, I figured out I had a reaction to pumpkin seeds. While I was a lacto-ovo vegetarian, I was eating loads of nuts and seeds, including pumpkin seeds, pumpkin seed butter and oil.

I felt hungry all the time. I had to always carry food with me, as I would get irritable and shaky if I didn't eat "on time"—both are typical symptoms of hypoglycemia and inability to maintain stable blood glucose. My gums were receding and, worst of all, my whole digestion was compromised. I had all the typical symptoms of dysbiosis (gut flora imbalance) and leaky gut with excess gas production in the upper and lower GI tract; bloating; indigestion; and many food sensitivities. I also began to have mood swings with a tendency toward depression.

That got really bad after giving birth to my son. Between the nutritional depletion associated with pregnancy and lactation, and the postpartum hormones, I was not feeling like myself. I was crying all the time and was chronically unhappy, to the point that my husband thought we should seek a psychiatrist's help. Of course, I didn't want that.

I knew something wasn't right, but I also knew it wasn't an anti-depression drug deficiency that I suffered from. I had to figure this one out on my own. I am stubborn like that. I knew myself and my body the best, and I was determined to solve the puzzle of my progressively deteriorating health.

To make things even more worrisome, in the last trimester of pregnancy when I did the screening test for gestational diabetes, I didn't pass it. That was a huge surprise, as I thought I was doing all things right for my body. I was a faithful vegetarian, lean and fit. Even when pregnant, I gained weight by the book. From the outside, I looked like the perfect pregnant woman, yet, inside, things were going downhill quite rapidly. Take to the heart this message: never judge a book by its cover and a person by their looks, as they both can be deceiving.

Interestingly enough, all those years—actually throughout my life—weight was never an issue for me. I was always lean, fit and physically active. But that didn't compensate for the excess sugar I was getting from my plant-based diet (from all the starches and grains, plus the tons of fruits—mind you, those were all whole foods). I simply ate more carbohydrates than my body could safely metabolize and that took a toll on my pancreas. I developed a degree of insulin resistance, which was amplified during pregnancy and manifested as gestational diabetes.

I was devastated, to say the least. I just couldn't believe it. Having the knowledge I have now, I do believe it and it all makes sense. Back then I couldn't understand, *how is it possible to be a vegetarian, eat whole foods, be physically active, never be overweight and get gestational diabetes?*

I began to test my blood sugar before and after meals, and cut back on the amount of carbs I ate. That helped. Today, I can safely consume 70 g of net carbs a day (although my average ranges from 30-50 g) and have well-controlled blood sugars.

The time when I embarked on the raw foods journey was also the time when I decided to make a career change. I was already living in the USA, and I enrolled into a Masters in Nutrition program. It made sense to dive deep into the science of healing with foods, as I was interested at a personal level and it had always been my passion.

So, my healing with foods quest blended with my new career path. What I learned from textbooks, I applied to my personal life and, later, with my patients when I worked for a major hospital in Miami, and with my private clients when I opened my own practice, Healing With Foods.

It took many trials before I figured out what I needed to do to get my health back and how to best help my clients do the same, using food and lifestyle as the main therapies. In fact, it took 10 more years; years when I went from raw vegan to eating healing, nourishing animal foods again. It was definitely not easy to go from being a vegetarian back to eating animal food. But, when "pain" is greater than a desire to live up to an ideology, the "pain wins" and change takes place.

I gave up being a vegetarian in exchange for healing my body.

At one of the integrative nutrition conferences I attended at the University of Miami, I learned about a supplements company that had done a lot of research in the gut health area. I started taking every webinar they had on gut dysfunction and further learned from everything I could get my hands, ears and eyes on. From courses to books to programs, I devoured them all. I began taking some gut healing supplements, and I was willing to add to my plant-based diet eggs and fermented dairy, mainly kefir.

For the first time, I had significant improvement. Finally something was working! I had about 50% improvement, but I was far from feeling like myself again. When I learned about elimination diets, I had an ALCAT food sensitivity test done, and I started to eliminate from my diet the foods I was sensitive to that where causing inflammation in my system. I was having a mild form of leaky gut where partially digested or undigested foods were entering my bloodstream and my immune system was fighting against the whole foods I was eating. The things that I was sensitive to were all healthy whole foods (figs, almonds, carrot, basil, coffee). Yep, that was the year I gave up coffee. Ah, it was hard, but you know what? I had another improvement in my symptoms. I was feeling 70% better.

About 1 year after my first elimination diet and taking gut healing supplements, I had no more improvement and some of the gut symptoms returned. The mood swings were getting worse; I was going head first towards depression (by that time I was about 1 year postpartum, which I'm sure had something to do with it too). Around this time, I came across Dr. Natasha Campbell McBride's work. It completely resonated with me. I applied for her training certification program to become a GAPS Certified Practitioner. I was accepted. I knew I wanted to learn more about her approach. I wanted to use it personally and, if it delivered as much as it promised, I was going to use it with my private clients as well.

When I attended the course with Dr. Natasha, I was still a lacto-ovo vegetarian. Her explanation of the gut-brain and the gut-body connection made so much sense, both common and pathophysiological. I dropped all the resistance; I understood that I had to incorporate animal foods back into my diet if I wanted to heal my body and my mind. My desire to heal was strong! I have no words to describe how strong. You can probably imagine, by then it had been a total of twenty years of trials and learning.

After 10 years on a plant-based diet, I embraced the healing power of animal foods.

Was it hard? Yes and no!

Did my body reject the animal fat or the meat? No!

Actually, my gut felt good when I had my first meat and bone broth. It was soothing to my gut.

Mentally, it was another story. I was trying not to think about the fact that I was eating flesh again, which I thought I would never go back to. I was willing to give this approach a fair try before I would cast my vote on it. I was mentally ready! It really was, and is, all a matter of mindset.

Before, when an acupuncturist suggested that I should add animal foods back into my diet, I rejected the idea vehemently. I wasn't ready!

I wasn't ill enough. I didn't struggle enough. The pain wasn't deep enough.

I didn't have the understanding of gut health as being the most important piece of the healing puzzle either.

I wasn't aware of the power that animal fat and protein play in nourishment and healing; thus, I couldn't make the change.

I learned that we humans make changes when we are aware of the need to change. I also learned that the most important catalyst for change is inner motivation.

We are motivated by pain, fear or desire.

- Pain, like I had: stomach pain, pain of pricking my fingers 10 times a day to monitor my blood sugar, pain of counting carbs, pain of being a depressed mom and wife.

- Fear, such as that of a person with cancer, fear of losing one's life, or fear of losing a leg or vision, as an uncontrolled diabetic may have.

- Desire, like that of body builders or ballerinas; they act on pure desire to perform or look a certain way.

It's human nature; it's either pain or pleasure that will motivate us to change.

Next let's take a look at some painful health statistics: The Status Quo.

THE STATUS QUO

Let's take a look at the modern, 21st century man.

As you probably know the picture of the "comfortable, modern, industrialized, computerized man, woman and children" is not very pretty. All you need to do the next time you are in a public place, such as a zoo or an amusement park, is look around and you'll see that most of the population, from children to adults, are overweight and obese.

According to the latest statistics released by the CDC (Center for Disease Control and Prevention), in the USA the percent of adults age 20 years and older that are overweight or obese is 70.7%. [7]

That's a staggering number!

The situation doesn't look too good either when we look at our adolescent and child population, who have a 20.6% obesity rate among 12-19 year-olds and 17.4% obesity rate in 6-11 year-olds children.

Obesity is a huge problem that is more than aesthetic. It comes with a big price: risk of disease.

Let's take a look at diabetes and autoimmune diseases, as they are linked to obesity and inflammation. They are diet and lifestyle related. If they are caused by something, they can be reverse by the same means.

It's a choice we all have!

According to a CDC report dated 2014, in the USA 29.1 million people currently have diabetes. That is approximately 1 in every 11 adults. 1 in 4 of these people are not even aware of having it. [8]

The picture is even worse when it comes to pre-diabetes; 86 million people have prediabetes. That means 1 in every 3 people is pre-diabetic. What is even more scary is that 9 out of 10 of these individuals are not even aware they are pre-diabetic. It is predicted that 15 to 30% of people that have prediabetes will develop diabetes within five years if they don't lose weight, and change their food and lifestyle.

I should perhaps clarify that prediabetes precedes diabetes. It occurs some-times for 15-20 years before it gets diagnosed as diabetes.

As you can see, the future of our nation doesn't look good at all.

Diabetes comes with enormous financial and personal costs. Currently, 245 billion dollars are spent on medical costs and lost wages for people with di-abetes. Let's take into consideration that the risk of death for a person with diabetes is 50% higher than for a person without diabetes. Some complications of diabetes include loss of vision, kidney failure with the need for dialysis, car-diovascular disease, dementia and Alzheimer's, along with loss of toes, feet and legs, leading to amputation.

According to the American Autoimmune Related Diseases Association [9], there are currently 50 million Americans diagnosed with an Autoimmune Disease (AD). AD is the #1 most popular health topic requested by callers to the Nation-al Women's Health Information Center.

> *"NIH estimates annual direct healthcare costs for AD to be in the range of $100 billion (source: NIH presentation by Dr. Fauci, NIAID). In comparison, cancer costs are $57 billion (source: NIH, ACS), and heart and stroke costs are $200 billion (source: NIH, AHA)."*[9]

An AD is a condition in which the immune system doesn't recognize the body's own tissues as safe. Thus, it triggers an immune response against the "self"— for example, against pancreatic tissues known in type 1 diabetes or against thyroid tissue known as Hashimoto's.

The purpose of sharing these statistics is not to overwhelm you, nor to instill fear in you. On the contrary, because we know "ignorance is not bliss," this knowledge may help you change in order to prevent these diseases or to reverse them if you are already afflicted.

My intention for writing this book is simple: when you are done reading this book, I want you to feel empowered, to gain knowledge and confidence, to believe in yourself, and to have the tools you need to take action. I will bring together traditional and ancient wisdom with the latest nutrition science. This information, together with your body's innate intelligence, will allow you to take full charge of your health, life, and happiness.

I will give you not only the "what and why," but also the "how to." These are the tools and the strategies I've been using personally and with my private clients for over one decade.

But first let's see if this book is for you.

WHO IS THIS BOOK FOR?

This Book Is For You If:

- you have diabetes or pre-diabetes, dyslipidemia, non-alcoholic fatty liver disease, inflammation, joint pain, headaches/migraines;

- you suffer from chronic fatigue, lack of energy, mood swings or cravings;

- you have a hard time losing weight or maintaining weight loss;

- you have gastrointestinal problems—whether it's constipation or diarrhea, gas, bloating, indigestion, or acid reflux;

- you have been diagnosed with an autoimmune condition, have asthma, allergies, or other inflammatory problems;

- you are proactive and would like to know how to support your body's health and prevent disease processes by using a whole food (low carb) approach;

- you would like to increase your mental and physical energy and performance;

- you would like to use a keto approach to "upgrade your biology," to learn how to become a "fat burner" and perform better in business and life;

- you wish to be in control of your hunger and food choices, to get rid of food cravings, and to be at peace with food;

- you feel overwhelmed and confused about the conflicting nutrition information out there, you feel frustrated or stuck and unable to take action, *"paralysis by analysis"*; and/or

- you heard about nutritional ketosis and ketogenic diet, but are not sure what those are, how they can help you, or how to begin your journey into the keto world.

Although I believe that anyone can benefit from reading this book, this book may not be for you if:

- you are healthy and fit;

- you are happy with your body and energy;

- you have a healthy relationship with food;

- you perform well mentally and physically; and/or

- you don't have a family history of diabetes, metabolic syndrome, obesity, cardiovascular disease, cancer, neurodegenerative conditions, etc.

Why change what's already working, right?

AWARENESS

PART 1:
FOOD AND ITS METABOLIC EFFECTS

Defining Food.

When you say food, when you think about food, what do you mean? What do you see with your mind's eye? I'm sure the meaning you give to this word "food" is as unique as you are. In fact, there are as many interpretations given to this word as there are people living on our planet.

Yet, somehow we need to define "food." Given that a big part of this book is focused on food, I feel it is extremely important for us to have the same understanding of "food."

With that being said, let's see what I mean when I say food. The short answer would be, *"whole foods."* But even this leaves room for interpretation.

I use the following criteria to sort foods that are available to us today:

1. **My great-grandmother and her grandmother would recognize it as food** (that takes us at least 200-300 years back). I often refer to this as traditional eating.

> Here, we tap into traditional wisdom. According to blogs.ancestry.com in the article "What did people eat in 1800s?" people ate mostly what they grew in their gardens or hunted locally. Some of the food items

mentioned in the article were corn, potato, beans, milk, butter, and meats such as pork, beef, bison and other game provided meats.

Before refrigeration was invented, food preservation was done by smoking, drying, and salting for meats and fermenting or storing in root cellars for vegetables.[1]

2. **If it comes in a package (box, jar, bag, etc.), the ingredients should be legible, pronounceable and there should be no more than 5-7 ingredients (preferably 1-3).**

My 6-year-old and I should be able to read and pronounce the ingredients. I shouldn't even participate in this test, as I majored in biochemistry, so I'm pretty good at reading and pronouncing chemicals, but keep in mind that we are talking about food here, not about food experiments. I hope you agree with me on this one. Don't allow the food industry to run chemistry experiments on you!

Let me give you an example or two of a food that may come in a package, yet is a whole food or is made from whole foods ingredients. Let's take as an example sardines in a can; Ingredients: sardines, water, sea salt-packed in a BPA free can (brand name Wild Planet). Similarly, coconut oil-comes in jar or BPA free container, and the only ingredient that's listed is organic, cold-pressed coconut oil. OK, one more example. Let's say you are looking for a snack such as a protein or granola bar. A great example would be Lara bars. Let's look at Cashew Cookies bar from their original line. It lists two ingredients: cashews and dates.

I think you get the point: find foods that are simple, made with pronounceable ingredients.

3. **The food is as close to its whole, unprocessed form as possible.**

There are foods today that are generally and widely accepted as food; yet, personally, I do not consider them "food" and I choose not to consume them, endorse them or recommend them to my clients.

These examples will help you understand why:

Let's take a look at grains, to see how the foods we find today in the supermarket made out of grains are highly processed, refined and void of nutrients. Thus, they do not deserve the qualification of food. What do we find made out of grains today? Some good examples are, baked goods (bagels, donuts, Danishes, etc.), pastries, cereals (dry or wet), bars, cookies, cakes, pastas and breads. Refined grain flour turned into even more refined and processed food-like substances.

"What about whole grains Mihaela, like brown rice, steel cut oats, quinoa?" I can hear you saying. Later in the gut and inflammation section, I will cover why grains, whole or refined, are inflammatory and gut damaging. If you wish to heal your gut, you may want to shy away from them.

4. **Food should mimic ancestral food.**

Would the food you eat be recognized by the ancestral man? I understand it's not easy to know exactly what humans roaming the earth 200,000 years ago, or more, ate. I'm sure it was varied and differed from region to region.

According to an article published in Nature, International Weekly Journal Of Science, the oldest humans (homo sapiens) lived approximately 195,000 year ago and were discovered in Africa.[2] It is said that Africa, and Ethiopia in particular, was the birthplace of humans.

With that in mind, let's see what they were possibly eating 200,000 years ago. The Great Rift Valley, a wide area of approximately 6000 km (3,700 mi) in length, stretches all the way from Asia to South Africa, and is the region we believe homo sapiens made their start before they ventured across the ocean and spread to other areas.[3] Looking at the landscape and what African tribes still living there today have access to, we can make an educated guess with respect to what they ate.

They had access to fresh and salt water (lakes, rivers and the sea), hence fish and seafood were part of their diet. This certainly provided them with a good source of protein and fat—the most important probably being the essential fatty acids (long chain omega-3 fats) which are our master anti-inflammatory fats and play a crucial role in fetal brain development, cardiovascular health and immune health, etc.

Hunting of animals roaming the coast of Africa was a practice the ancestral man engaged in. It is certain that, upon catching an animal, the ancestral man wasted none of it. From skin to organs, the prey was used entirely.[3] Similarly, when I was growing up only 40 years ago in Communist Romania, my parents used all the parts of the animals, and they still do to this day. It is believed that the ancestral man used even the blood of the hunt. Yes, even the stomach and the intestines were washed, cleaned properly and used in various forms. The stomach was used as a storage container for fat. It may come as a surprise to you, but the most nutrient dense animal foods are actually the organ meat and not the muscle meat.[4]

What about plant foods? Did the ancestral man eat plant foods at all? We know that grains and legumes were introduced late in human history, about 10,000 years ago with the agricultural era. An article published in National Geographic Magazine, The Evolution of Diet, states:

> "Until agriculture was developed around 10,000 years ago, all humans got their food by hunting, gathering, and fishing. As farming emerged, nomadic hunter-gatherers gradually were pushed off prime farmland, and eventually they became limited to the forests of the Amazon, the arid grasslands of Africa, the remote islands of Southeast Asia, and the tundra of the Arctic.

Today only a few scattered tribes of hunter-gatherers remain on the planet."[5]

That's not to say that the ancestral man had no plant food at all to their diet. Humans can consume any edible, non-toxic plant. It seems that tubers, berries and other local seasonal fruits were consumed as they were available. It is worth mentioning that the tubers that were found in the wild (unlike the potatoes known to us today) were very low in starch (the easy high insulinogenic carbohydrate we'll be talking about throughout the book) and were much higher in fibers that act as prebiotic-food for the gut microbes. So, it is assumed that those foods didn't serve as much as an energy source, but rather a source of fermentable fibers for the health of the human gut flora, which, as we will see later, is essential for good digestion, gut and immune system health.[3]

To summarize it, the ancestral man had to acquire their food in a hard way. The food was wild, local, and seasonal, and whether it was animal or plant food, it was rather scarce and it was as nature provided it: not processed not packaged, without serving size or nutrition facts.

Now, if I was to take all these criteria and lump them together, food:

• does not come in boxes and packages in an unrecognizable form to someone that lived 300 years ago (e.g. cereals, chips, candies, pasta, bagels, flour, juice, etc.);

• is made of a few simple pronounceable ingredients;

• is grown locally and consumed seasonally;

• is both animal and plant with minimal processing and involves natural preservation techniques;

• differs greatly from region to region and season to season; and

• has traits of ancestral and traditional eating.

Food: Beyond Calories, Macronutrients and Pleasure.

Often, when we talk about food, we think about its caloric value (the calories we attribute to food). We think in terms of the macronutrients (carbohydrates, protein and fat) or the micronutrients (vitamins and minerals), the antioxidants and phytonutrients we obtain from consuming it. And, of course, we all associate food with pleasure. We often say, *"I love sweets"* or *"I love salty foods."*

These are all true and valid food associations, yet food is far more than calories, nutrients or pleasure. Food is information. Food has an epigenetic, hormonal and drug-like effect.

Food, Genes and Epigenetics.

Food is information to your genetic make-up. Food helps you write the script of your health and life.

Although we all inherit our genetic material from our ancestors, our genes are not our destiny. According to the new and emerging field of epigenetics ("above" genetics), we now know that factors from our environment have the ability to change the way our genes are expressed. Food and other modifiable lifestyle factors are acting upon our genes, are above or "pressing on," meaning that they override the genes, hence they dictate how they express themselves.

In other words, you may inherit a gene that predisposes you to developing, for example, diabetes. Let's say in your family, your mother or your father and some other close relatives have been diagnosed with diabetes, so it is expected that at some point in time you will develop diabetes as well. However, the way you live your life, your lifestyle, which includes food, as well as exercise, stress management, your thoughts and beliefs, sleep, smoking, alcohol, drugs, supplements, etc. will strongly determine whether you will or will not develop diabetes.

Having the gene for diabetes doesn't automatically mean you will have diabetes. The environment plays a big role in it.

What makes our environment? Internal and external factors.

Out of all the environmental factors that "press" on our genes, our "mind," the food we eat, the water we drink and the air we breathe are the most powerful epigenetic agents.

You think all the time, consciously and subconsciously, so your thoughts act as a powerful medicine or poison. As this book is mostly about food, I will not spend much time explaining the power of the mind in health and healing. For an in depth look at the power of beliefs in healing, I highly recommend the book "Power Of The Mind In Health And Healing" by Keith Holden, M.D.

The quality of the air also matters, as we breathe all the time. Toxic air is a powerful epigenetic agent. Breath work is also used in health and healing. My favorite breathing techniques are the nasal breathing, the Buteyko method. You can learn more about it at www.buteyko.com. Another breathing technique I personally like and use is the Wim Hoff Method, which you can find at www.wimhofmethod.com.

The same goes for water. In fact, we can survive longer without food than we can without water, so drinking clean, pure water is also a big contributing factor in health and healing. Look into investing in a good water filtration system. I recommend checking the Environmental Working Group site for their free water filtration systems buying guide, www.ewg.org.

These are all things we take for granted, but we should probably reevaluate that.

Since this book is about food, let's see how the food you choose to eat throughout your lifetime can strengthen the "bad" genes and facilitate the development of disease or, on the contrary, how food can prevent the "bad" genes from expressing and you can live a long healthy happy life.

Let's go back to the diabetes example. If you inherited the diabetes gene and you choose to eat a diet made of processed refined foods, high in carbohydrates, soft drinks and sweets, you exponentially increase your risk of developing diabetes. The very food you choose to eat strengthens the diabetes gene and facilitates its expression.

"Genes are loading the gun, but you through your choices pull the trigger." You are the one that makes a choice each and every time you take a bite of food or a sip of a beverage. Choose wisely! Use food as medicine, not as poison, because food is information for your genes. Food helps you write the script of your health and life.

Food, Hormones and Metabolism.

In this section we'll see how food interacts with the hormones that regulate energy metabolism and how that affects your weight and metabolic health. You will understand why looking at food as "calories" is a rather simplistic and incomplete way of talking about food. Often in my conversations with friends or family members I hear them say, *"You can eat that, it doesn't have calories,"* or *"This is high in calories. I won't eat it."*

It's time that you stop worrying about the calories in food, and you look at food more like you would look at a prescription "hormone."

First let me introduce the hormones that regulate energy balance:

- INSULIN: the master storage hormone

- GLUCAGON: the master mobilization hormone

How does food interact with these hormones?

Different macronutrients interact with different hormones and that translates into different metabolic effects. This food-hormone interaction is especially relevant when it comes to weight loss and the management of metabolic disorders, such as type II diabetes, polycystic ovarian syndrome (PCOS), metabolic syndrome, non-alcoholic fatty liver disease and dyslipidemia.

What are macronutrients?

Macro means big or large. Macronutrients are the nutrients we find in food in large amounts. There are three macronutrients: carbohydrate, protein and fat.

When it comes to calories, each one of these has a specific energetic value. See Table 1.

What is far more important, however, is the hormonal response each one of the macronutrients elicits in the body upon ingestion.

MACRONUTRIENT	ENERGETIC VALUE (CALORIES/GRAM)
Carbohydrate	4
Protein	4
Fat	9
Alcohol*	7

Table 1

*Alcohol is not a macronutrient, but it's worth mentioning as it is part of most people's food and lifestyle.

Carbohydrates and Insulin.

In Part 3 we will see exactly which foods contain "insulinogenic" carbohydrates, as not all carbs are created equal. But now it is time to introduce the star of this book, the star that runs the show of most chronic degenerative conditions known to humans today: INSULIN.

Insulin is a storage hormone, a growth hormone and a pro-inflammatory hormone.

To understand the relationship between carbohydrates and insulin, let's just say that all carbohydrates found in the foods we eat (except for fiber) are ultimately absorbed in the bloodstream as simple sugars, with the most prevalent one being glucose. Glucose is then used as an energy source immediately or stored as glycogen and fat for later use by the cells of our body. For that to happen, glucose needs to get from the blood to inside the cells, and that requires the hormone insulin. Insulin is a hormone produced by the pancreas, a gland that sits inside the abdominal cavity. In the absence of insulin, glucose remains "trapped" in the blood, where it reaches high levels and becomes toxic.

Type I diabetes, for example, is a disease caused by the absence of insulin. This is a life-threatening condition if not treated (with insulin). A type I diabetic has to know exactly how much carbohydrates they consume in order for them to calculate the exact amount of insulin needed to assist with the transfer of the glucose from the blood to the cells.

For those of us who have a "working" pancreas that produces insulin "on demand," we don't have to think about how much insulin our pancreas has to secrete to accommodate the carbs we eat. However, it pays off to think about how many carbohydrates we eat, because, as we'll see throughout this book, too many carbs and too much insulin come at a high health cost.

This is one instance in which "less is more!" Less carbs and less insulin, it turns out, to be good. Let me clarify: insulin in itself is not bad. Too much insulin in the blood (hyperinsulinemia) can be a problem. Hyperinsulinemia over time leads to insulin resistance and that is at the root cause of obesity and metabolic disorders. In the next section, The Three Common Factors in Chronic Disease, I will explain in greater detail what insulin resistance is. For now, let's try to understand insulin and its functions.

Insulin's number one job is to keep glucose in our blood at safe levels. Too much glucose in the blood (hyperglycemia) is a "toxic" metabolic state, seen in pre-diabetes and uncontrolled diabetes. The way insulin helps us maintain normal levels of glucose in the blood is by exerting a storage function. Insulin is a storage hormone that helps us save energy from food, in times of "feast" for times of "famine." It served us extremely well in the Paleolithic era and up to 10,000 years ago, before the agriculture era, when food was scarce and was lacking carbohydrates for the most part.

Today, when food is abundant, is made predominantly of carbohydrates (which are also highly refined), and is easily obtained (doesn't require much effort to fill up a shopping cart with packages of convenient "food"), insulin's great storage ability may work against us. Why doesn't insulin just stop saving energy? It can't! One thing is sure: we can't change the way insulin works! We can't tell our body not to produce insulin, and not to store energy when too much food is available. In fact, if we pause for a second and look at this scenario, we can see that the problem is not with the insulin, the problem is with too much food that triggers insulin secretion. There is just too much glucose in the blood that needs to be pushed out into the cells by insulin. Insulin just performs its job. The logical solution to this problem is to control the amount and the type of food we eat—mainly to cut back on the high carbohydrate foods. By doing this, we have less demand for insulin, so we store less, and we stay lean and metabolically healthy.

Let's look at how insulin keeps normal blood sugar levels. *See Diagram 1 on the next page.* When we eat a meal that's high in "insulinogenic" carbohydrates, and there is too much glucose in the blood, the insulin makes possible for some of it to be used as energy by the working muscles and brain (according to the body's needs for energy), some is stored as glycogen (inside the liver and muscles) and, when that storage gets filled up, the rest of the glucose is stored as fat inside the adipose tissue (de novo lipogenesis). It's worth mentioning that if the glycogen storage is very limited, it can only go up to 2000 calories while the fat storage is virtually limitless, it goes well over 40,000 calories, even for a lean individual.[42]

When insulin stops doing its job (either because of insulin resistance or due to lack of insulin secretion by the pancreas), you will have elevated blood sugar levels and you may be diagnosed with diabetes or pre-diabetes.

The logical step to prevent all of these issues (hyperglycemia, hyperinsulinemia, and de novo lipogenesis) is to simply eat less insulinogenic carbs!

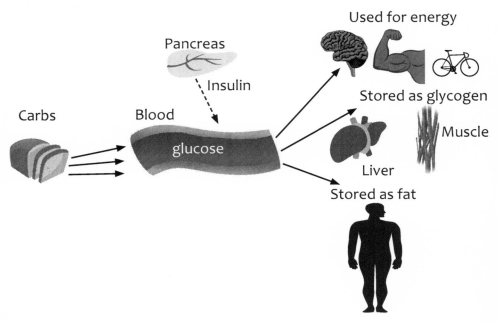

Diagram #1: Carbohydrate absorbtion and metabolism

Proteins and Glucagon.

Eating protein, doesn't cause a spike in blood sugar, hence it doesn't require insulin to be metabolized. On the contrary protein stimulates glucagon release.

Glucagon is the "brother" hormone. Both insulin and glucagon are secreted in the pancreas, by different cells. Insulin is secreted by the beta pancreatic cells, while glucagon is secreted by the alpha pancreatic cells. However, they have opposite metabolic effects.

Insulin is the energy storage hormone; glucagon is the energy wasting hormone.

They are both in charge of maintaining normal blood glucose levels. Insulin is called in when there is too much sugar in the blood while glucagon is called in when there is not enough. They are like shift workers; they work in the same place for the same organization, generate the same end product (normal blood glucose), but in very different ways and they don't meet.

Later we'll get more into how glucagon helps maintain normal blood glucose levels, but for the purpose of understanding the hormonal effect of macronutrients, let's just keep in mind that the macronutrient protein stimulates glucagon release.

Protein can be insulinogenic.

When protein is consumed in excess, especially in the context of low carbohydrate intake, it has an insulin stimulating effect as well—about half that of carbohydrates. If we were to assign a value of 1 to the insulin response to carbohydrate consumption, then we would assign a value of 0.5 to the insulin response to protein. You may ask how is this possible? There are some amino acids (called gluconeogenic) that are used by the liver as a substrate to produce glucose in a process called gluconeogenesis (gluco=sugar, neo=new, genesis= production or creation). In other words, the liver is producing glucose from non-glucose sources—in this case from amino acids. This effect is primarily seen in people with insulin resistance, type I and type II diabetics and is amplified in a context of low carbohydrate intake.[43]

Marty Kendall in his blog www.optimizingnutrition.com gets well into the details of the gluconeogenic and insulinogenic effect of protein, and he created a food insulin index that is a great resource to use, especially if your goal is managing diabetes with food. He classifies foods by taking into account both the insulinogenic carbohydrates and the gluconeogenic protein content. He developed a formula that helps evaluate the insuliogenic effect of a meal.

(Total grams of Insulinogenic Carbohydrates X 1) + (grams of Protein X 0.56) = Insulin Load

IC (g) + Protein (g) X 0.56 = IL

- *Insulinogenic carbohydrates (IC) are total carbohydrates minus fiber, they are also known as Net Carbohydrates (NC)*

- 1 is the factor assigned to insulin response to IC consumption

- 0.56 is the factor assigned to insulin response to protein consumption, as about half of the amino acids can convert into sugar

- Insulin load is the total amount of insulin required to metabolize the glucose from a meal

Most people seem to achieve good glycemic control and to maintain nutritional ketosis at an IL around 125. You will have to see what your magic number is.

If you have difficulty managing blood sugars, despite the fact that you follow a low carbohydrate eating plan, begin to pay attention to the amount of protein you consume at each meal as well as your individual glycemic response to protein. There appears to be individual variations with regards to blood sugar and insulin response to protein consumption, just as there is to carbohydrates.

In the section Protein 101, we discuss "Protein, How Much is Too Much," and we'll talk more about the relevance of excess protein consumption, and how to calculate your protein needs.

A well-designed low carbohydrate nutrition protocol is not high in protein; it's low to moderate in protein and high in fat. In fact a better way to describe it would be adequate protein. If protein is good, more is not better.

Thus, excess protein consumption is not necessarily a good thing. More about this in Protein 101.

Fats are Hormonally Neutral.

Fats do not induce insulin nor a glucagon response. So, from a metabolic hormonal perspective, fats are neutral. In fact, fat consumption mimics fasting.

To understand fat in relationship to metabolic hormones, let's first have a look at what happens hormonally when we fast.

In the absence of food (fasting), when the body's need for energy is no longer met by an external supply, the body taps into its reserves. I briefly mentioned before that when we eat (primarily carbs), we store energy in two forms and in two separate reservoirs: *glycogen* (stored carbohydrates) in the liver and in the muscles and *fat* inside the adipose tissue, both under the skin as well as inside the abdominal cavity.[52] See Diagram 2.

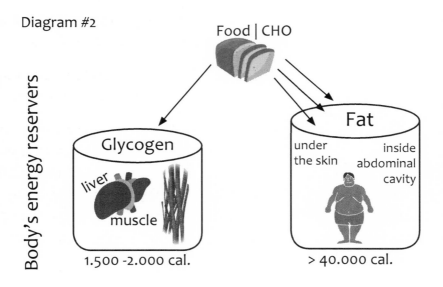

Diagram #2

During an overnight fast, a prolonged fast or prolonged exercising, the body gets its energy first by breaking down the glycogen reserves. The glycogen from the liver is converted back into glucose and is sent into the blood to maintain normal glycemia and supply energy for the entire body. The muscles are a bit selfish so they keep all the glycogen for themselves and supply energy only to the working muscles. It is estimated that a 70 kg man, stores only 18 hours of fuel supply as glycogen, compared with a two month supply of fat. [52]This energy reservoir is pretty small, and rapidly empties out. It varies from individual to individual, and activity level is a big determining factor to how fast glycogen is used up. When this happens, and food still doesn't come to supply energy, the body goes to the second, larger reservoir: the fat.

It begins to mobilize fat and to turn it into energy. Some free fatty acids are used directly as energy sources by the muscles; however, the main energy derived from fat is in the form of ketone bodies. Fat conversion into ketones is happening in the liver, inside the mitochondria (the energy generators of the cell), via a process called beta oxidation.

While glycogen is converted back into glucose, fat is converted into ketones. Ketone bodies enter the blood stream and supply energy to the body including the brain. This is very important as the brain can't use fatty acid as energy.

As the body begins to burn fat for energy, it also turns on the backup system that helps maintain normal levels of glucose in the blood, gluconeogenesis.

This is a built-in survival mechanism that allows the body to always supply energy to the cells that rely exclusively on glucose for their function, such as the red blood cells, retinas, and liver cells. The body uses glucogenic amino acids and the glycerol bone from fatty acids metabolism to generate its own glucose for the glucose dependent tissues. What does this mean? It means you can go for a very long time without food or carbohydrates, and supply energy for your body from your own reserves.

This is indeed a true state of adaptation to the unfriendly environment our ancestors were exposed to while evolving here on earth, when food was scarce, difficult to obtain and had a completely different macronutrient distribution than what we see today.

All of the above described metabolic pathways are carefully orchestrated by hormones.

When fasting, insulin levels drop, while glucagon and the other counter regulatory hormones (adrenalin, noradrenalin, cortisol, human growth hormone) are rising. These hormones facilitate maintenance of normal blood sugar levels, as well as energy generation from fat stores.

Teaser: another interesting process that takes place during fasting is that the body goes into a cellular cleansing, which *"is a regulated orderly process of breaking down and recycling cellular compounds when there's no longer enough energy to sustain them."*[10] We will go into this process in the Fasting 101 section.

Now that we have an understanding of what happens hormonally and metabolically in the absence of food, let's have a look at fat and its hormonal effects on the body.

Consumption of fat alone does not elicit an insulin response, as it is hormonally neutral. Hence, we see a very similar metabolic and hormonal effect to that seen during fasting.

It's safe to say that you "can eat fat to burn fat" and "that carbs are actually fat in disguise," because when we eat carbs, we store them as fat.

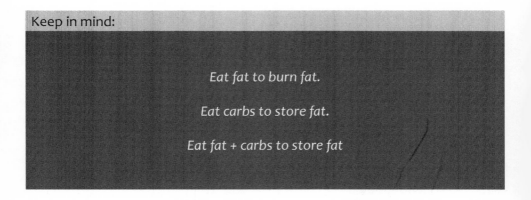

Keep in mind:

Eat fat to burn fat.

Eat carbs to store fat.

Eat fat + carbs to store fat

Thus, when you begin to consume fat as your primary source of energy while restricting carbohydrates and eating moderate amounts of protein, you switch your "modern day metabolism," which runs on carbs, back to the "ancestral metabolism," the one that runs on fat (and ketones). This translates into weight loss (fat loss), improved blood sugar management, reversal of fatty liver, as well as other traits of metabolic syndrome, reduction in inflammation, and "endless" energy—both mental and physical.

> You can't burn both substrates at the same time.
>
> *To burn fat, you can't eat FAT and CARBS together!*
>
> *Swap bread and butter for broccoli and butter.*

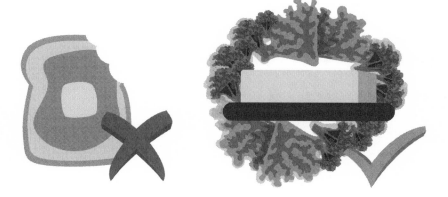

Do not worry if you feel at a loss right now. Before the end of the book you will be very clear about what you can eat to burn fat so you can reap all the metabolic benefits that are associated with it. You will know very well how to put together a well-designed low carbohydrate, moderate protein and high fat meal plan, to heal and to thrive.

PART 2:
THE THREE COMMON FACTORS
IN CHRONIC DISEASE

How We Get Sick.

Understanding how we get sick is as important as understanding how we stay healthy. It helps both with prevention, as well as reversal, of disease.

In this part of the book, I will take some time to explain the three common factors seen today in all chronic degenerative conditions: insulin resistance, chronic global inflammation and leaky gut.

Please understand, it's never only one factor that leads to disease in the body; usually it is multifactorial and multidimensional. Although food is the center piece of this book, I'd like to reinforce the complexity of the matter and to mention stress in here. Stress is always one of the elements involved in disease processes. Stress acts as an accelerating factor. Keep this in mind as you go through this part of the book, as I don't want you to get the impression that these three factors are the only ones leading to diseases. That would be far from the truth.

Why these three and not more or others? Because they all respond to the same dietary intervention: elimination of insulinogenic carbohydrates. Three seemingly separate factors, one dietary intervention, and a broad spectrum of health benefits.

Why do I take the time to talk about this rather than just give you the healing protocols?

I believe that, in order to make a change, you must first understand WHY you need to change, and then learn the rationale behind it. We are the only living beings on this planet with a brain that allows us to reach conclusions based on logic and hard data (information). Let's then use our powerful brains to make informed, educated choices.

I believe that *"Knowledge Is Power."* You must know and understand first; only then you will take action. That's the recipe for success. Because, when you understand it, and act on it, you own the decision to make that change, and that is when you are most likely to embrace it as a lifelong approach. There is a big difference between me telling you to do something and you coming to the realization that you need to do that thing. I could just tell you, *"Do this and you'll lose weight, reverse diseases and have your life back,"* but I won't.

When the need to change comes from within, when it is based on knowledge and on a clear understanding of how the body works, chances are you'll embrace it as a life-style transformation, not as a temporary fix.

This next part will be a bit more technical. I will try to keep it as simple as possible. I encourage you to take the time to understand it before you jump to the action taking or the "Now That You Know, What Do You Do!" section.

Once you understand WHY, the HOW becomes 10X easier.

Factor #1

Insulin, Hyperinsulinemia, and Insulin Resistance.

Insulin

Although we already talked about insulin, I feel we need to spend a bit of time to introduce it properly. According to the Merriam Webster Dictionary, insulin is *"a protein pancreatic hormone secreted by the beta cells of the islets of Langerhans that is essential especially for the metabolism of carbohydrates and the regulation of glucose levels in the blood and that, when insufficiently produced, results in diabetes mellitus."* [6]

This vital hormone was discovered in 1922 by Dr. Frederick Banting, who was awarded the Nobel Prize one year later for his discovery.

Insulin performs a few jobs in the body, but probably the most important is glycemic control: making sure that when glucose levels rise in the blood (mainly upon consuming carbohydrate-containing foods) they are brought back down to "safe levels." This is very important because elevated blood glucose levels are not safe. In fact, they are very damaging to all cells in the body. Hyperglycemia is a toxic state.

Under normal circumstances, we hold 5-10 grams of glucose in our bloodstream at any given time, which is the equivalent of one to two teaspoons. [21] Our body was designed to protect us against the harmful effects of excess glucose by responding with insulin. When sugar enters the bloodstream—such as immediately after consuming a meal, e.g. bagel with cream cheese, jam, and orange juice; cereal with milk; or a big bowl of fruits—insulin is released from the pancreas and will facilitate the transfer of excess glucose from the blood into the cells to be used as an energy source. Some of the free glucose coming from dietary sources is used to replenish glycogen stores (if they are depleted), and the rest goes to be stored as fat inside the adipose tissue. For a visual representation, please refer to Diagram 1 on page 46.

With the type of food we eat in the modern era, insulin's glycemic management often translates into fat storage. The process of converting excess glucose into fatty acids is known as de novo lipogenesis.

novo = new, lipo = fat, genesis = production

Often you will hear me saying that carbs are fats in disguise.

Let's see what else insulin does in the body:

- Insulin participates in hunger and satiety regulation by stimulating centers in the hypothalamus (a part of the brain).

- Insulin is an anabolic hormone and is essential for the growth of many tissues and organs. We have anabolic and catabolic hormones. An example of a catabolic hormone is glucagon. The balance of the two is crucial for the health and maintenance of our body (breakdown and repair). Too much insulin can cause excessive growth—primarily of the fat cells, but other cells as well, like cancer cells and epithelial cells that line blood vessels.

- Insulin also plays a crucial role in regulation/counter-regulation of other hormones, such as glucagon, adrenaline, and cortisol.

Hyperinsulinemia & Insulin Resistance (IR).

First let's define these terms.

Hyperinsulinemia means elevated levels of insulin in the blood.

Hyper = elevated/high, insulin = the hormone, emia = blood.

Insulin resistance, just as the name implies, is a state in which the cells of the body become resistant to the actions of insulin. The exact mechanism by which insulin facilitates the transfer of the glucose from the bloodstream, inside the cells of the body, is very complex and is beyond the scope of this book. Think of insulin as a messenger that communicates with the cell receptors, it lets them know that glucose is coming; hence, the cell needs to open the gates and to send carriers from inside the cells out to the gates and transport the glucose inside. It's a well-orchestrated flow of events. When a person becomes IR, this entire process is impaired and the body responds by producing more insulin in order to keep this flow going and to maintain normal levels of blood glucose.

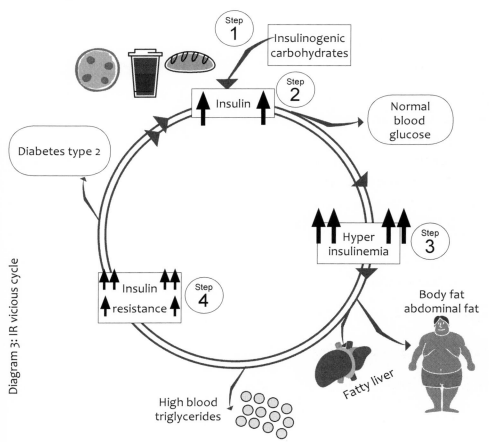

Diagram 3: IR vicious cycle

In an insulin-resistant person, we often find elevated levels of insulin (hyperinsulinemia) with normal blood sugar levels, meaning the body works harder to maintain normal blood sugar levels by sending more messengers; it produces more and more insulin to get the same end result. That comes at a high cost, which is paid by the pancreatic cells. The pancreas gets exhausted from doing all the hard work and, eventually, it stops producing insulin. This is usually the most advanced stage of the uncontrolled type II diabetic, which is managed with insulin injections and oral hypoglycemic drugs. The good news is that if the pancreas still has any working beta cells left, by eliminating insulinogenic carbs, it can regain some of its insulin secretion function and the person may go off insulin.

Common scenarios we see in type II diabetes

- Elevated insulin and elevated blood sugar. When the person is highly IR and the pancreas is working hard to maintain normal glycemia, but it fails.

- Increased body fat reserves, subcutaneous and visceral fat (abdominal obesity).

- Increased deposition of fat in the liver (nonalcoholic fatty liver).

- Increased levels of fats in the blood (high triglycerides).

- Decreased insulin and elevated blood sugar. When the pancreas goes on strike, it can't produce enough insulin. This is usually seen in a very advanced type II diabetic and insulin is then prescribed to manage their blood sugars.

IR doesn't happen overnight. It takes years or decades for this to happen. The more carbohydrates a person consumes, the more hyperinsulinemic they become. The more insulin the body is exposed to, the more it becomes resistant to its actions. The more insulin resistant, the greater the need for insulin to maintain normal blood sugars (euglycemia).[11]

It's a vicious cycle. See Diagram 3. The IR cycle is fueled by the intake of insulinogenic carbs (step 1). To stop this vicious cycle and to reverse IR and its metabolic effects (steps 2-4) we need to intervene at step 1 by removing the insulinogenic carbs.

Hyperinsulinemia and IR are directly caused by diet and lifestyle choices. Hence, early detection and intervention have the potential to change the course of the metabolic disease process.

It is like building a Lego®. You know the two-in-one Legos®? Recently, we bought one of those for my son. We could build either a helicopter or a boat. Depending on what we wanted to build, we had to choose the appropriate instruction manual and the pieces to build the desired Lego® structure. Well, when it comes to our life we have two possible outcomes: a *"healthy, happy, vibrant life"* or a *"diseased, in pain and frustrated life."* The Lego® pieces to build our life are basically food and lifestyle. You can choose the food and lifestyle that helps you build a *"healthy, happy, vibrant life,"* or the food and lifestyle that will lead to the other option, a *"diseased, in pain and frustrated life."* Ultimately the choice is yours.

If you are reading this book, you are already looking at the instruction manual that will lead to a *"healthy, happy, vibrant life."* Congratulations! Keep reading. This book provides you with the Lego® pieces you need to build the *"happy, healthy, vibrant life."*

So far, we talked about insulin and its functions plus the state of hyperinsulinemia and insulin resistance. We've covered how carbohydrates are the main macronutrient responsible for triggering an insulin response, and how over-consumption of insulinogenic carbohydrates leads to hyperinsulinemia and insulin resistance.

Let's have a look now at how we can measure hyperinsulinemia and insulin resistance, since early detection is the key to preventing the development of metabolic diseases.

How do we measure hyperinsulinemia and IR?

There are multiple ways in which we can measure our body's response to insulin and insulin resistance. The golden standard is a method called the insulin clamp, which is a rather invasive, expansive, and time-consuming method.

One of the more widely used methods in clinical practice that I would like to mention is called Homeostasis Model Assessment of Insulin Resistance (HOMA-IR). This is based on a formula which uses fasting blood glucose in millimoles multiplied by fasting blood insulin divided by 22.5. The smaller the number, the less insulin resistant a person is.

$$\text{HOMA-IR} = \frac{\text{FastingBS(mMol) x Fasting Insulin}}{22.5}$$

This is a laboratory test your doctor can order, or you can use the formula below to calculate your HOMA-IR score.

Let's take an example and see how you can use this:

Fasting BS: 87 mg/dl or (4.8 mMol)

Fasting insulin: 3.2 uU/ml

To convert mg/dl to mMol we divide by 18.

87:18=4.8

(4.8X3.2):22.5 = 0.68-no sign of IR

OR

Fasting BS 87 mg/dl or (4.8 mmol)

Fasting Insulin 13 uU/ml

(4.8X13):22.5 =2.77- indicative of IR

Look at this method of assessing IR as an approximation, like an early yellow, orange or red flag indicating possible insulin resistance.[56]

Another test worth mentioning here is HbA1C (Hemoglobin A1C).

HbA1C is a blood test which measures the amount of glucose that attaches to the surface of your red blood cells and gives an indication about the average blood sugar for approximately 3 months, which is the lifespan of red blood cells.

Looking at both HbA1C value and HOMA-IR will give you a more complete picture. They serve as early indicators of the state of metabolic imbalance induced by overconsumption of carbohydrates.

Below you'll see the criteria used by the American Diabetes Association to diagnose diabetes and prediabetes, based on HbA1C.[49]

Diagram #4 - HbA1C classification

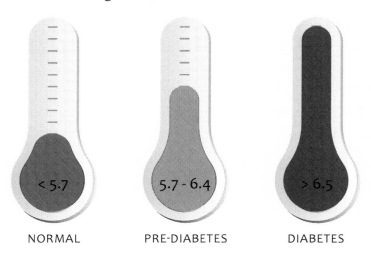

| < 5.7 | 5.7 - 6.4 | > 6.5 |
| NORMAL | PRE-DIABETES | DIABETES |

One other way to detect early patterns of hyperinsulinemia and IR is Dr. Joseph's Kraft insulin assay, a test similar to the oral glucose tolerance test (OGTT).

> *The oral glucose tolerance test (OGTT) is a standardized test used to diagnose a person with diabetes or impaired glucose tolerance (IGT). This is performed at a laboratory site and it measures fasting blood sugar, as well as the glucose curve over a period of 3 hours after ingesting 75 mg of glucose.*

Dr. Kraft is known as the father of the insulin assay and he's a proponent of the theory that diabetes is a vascular disease. His work is summarized in the book he wrote: *Diabetes Epidemic & You.*

His test is the most comprehensive; it provides a complete picture of glucose and insulin, both after fasting and post-administering 100 mg of glucose (75 mg works just as well). It's a curve of insulin and glucose after fasting and over a period of 5 hours, while OGTT is a curve of only glucose. HMO it's only a snapshot of fasting insulin and blood glucose. The table below shows a comparison of the common tests used to assess glycemic control.

	Insulin	Glucose	Fasting	Over time 3-5 hours	Average
Kraft's Insulin Assay	X	X	X	X	
OGTT		X	X	X	
HOMA-IR	X	X	X		
HbA1C		X			X

Dr. Kraft's test is able to detect very early signs of poor glycemic control, or early diabetes. It shows that a person may have a normal glucose tolerance test result, but, when we look at their insulin results, we see that in order to have normal blood glucose levels the person responds with high levels of insulin, a state of hyperinsulinemia which precedes insulin resistance. This serves as an early indicator of diabetes.[11] It's a much more sensitive test than OGTT, HbA1C, or HOMA-IR. By knowing the insulin response in relationship to glucose consumed, a person can take proactive measures and prevent the full onset of diabetes simply by changing their food and lifestyle choices.

Dr. Kraft confirmed and standardized his measurements using 14,384 subjects of all ages. He described 5 distinct insulin patterns.[17]

- Pattern I is considered normal. It is called "euinsulinemia."

- Pattern II, III, and IV are abnormal insulin responses indicative of hyperinsulinemia, also called diabetes "in-situ."

- Pattern V, consistent with type 1 diabetes and loss of beta cell function seen in advanced type II diabetes.

Now I know that this information is dry and it can be hard to grasp, but your doctor will get the meaning of it. That's why I created a chart for you with all these lab tests, so you can take it to your doctor and ask him to run some of these tests to help you assess your metabolic health and to determine your risk for developing diabetes. Even if you have already been diagnosed with diabetes, you can still benefit from some of these tests. With them, you will be able to assess how your body responds to dietary intervention, especially if you are going to implement the metabolic reset protocol (MRP), which will be discussed later.

Glycemic Lab Tests and Their Interpretation		
Fasting insulin	<5	
Fasting BS	<100	Ideally: 70-80
HMOA–IR	1 or less	
HbA1C	<5.3	
Kraft's Insulin assay	Aim for pattern I	

How Being Proactive vs. Reactive Can Benefit You.

If you want to be proactive—even if you don't think you may be at risk for developing diabetes or another metabolic disorder; even if you are lean and fit—I suggest periodically you run some of these tests. Knowledge is power and ignorance is not bliss. I'm the perfect example of a lean, fit person that had glycemic control issues.

I never had a weight problem and I was always active, yet during pregnancy I didn't pass the gestational diabetes screening test. It turns out I was building the Lego® of gestational diabetes with what I considered at the time to be healthy food. If I didn't have the test done, I would've never known until things got much worse. Because I knew, I was able to make changes in my food and lifestyle and stop the progression of the disease.

The earlier you find out that things are not going in the right direction and you take action to stop the snowball effect, the faster you will bounce out of it, or prevent the onset of a disease.

Why are hyperinsulinemia & insulin resistance dangerous?

I just used 1770 words explaining hyperinsulinemia and insulin resistance. It must be for a good reason, right?

Hyperinsulinemia and the more advanced state, insulin resistance are both major contributing factors to the development of metabolic disorders, the two most prevalent ones being type 2 diabetes and metabolic syndrome.

Metabolic syndrome is a cluster of conditions, which, when put together, drastically increase the risk of developing cardiovascular disease. To be diagnosed with metabolic syndrome one must have at least 3 of the 5 metabolic risk factors.

The five risk factors are: elevated blood pressure, elevated fasting blood sugar, increased abdominal obesity or waist circumference, abnormal lipid panel with low HDL, and elevated triglycerides levels. Some risk factors are different for women than they are for men.

For details, see the table below. Adapted from the NIH website. [44]

Metabolic Risk Factors	Female	Male
Waistline	>35 inches	>40 inches
High Blood Pressure	= or > 130/85	= or > 130/85
High Fasting Blood Sugar	> 100	> 100
High Triglycerides	> 150	> 150
Low HDL	<50	<40

Other hyperinsulinemic and IR related conditions worth mentioning are poly-cystic ovarian syndrome (PCOS), prediabetes, fatty liver (non-alcoholic fatty liver), overweight and obesity. It may come as a surprise to you, but even can-cer is a metabolic disorder that has hyperinsulinemia and IR as its root cause; so do Alzheimer's disease and other neurodegenerative diseases.

Since hyperinsulinemia and IR are at the core of metabolic disorders, and are diet induced, it's correct to say that metabolic diseases are diet and lifestyle in-duced as well. Hence, we can prevent them and reverse them if we change the true cause: diet and lifestyle. If we were to refer again to the Lego® example, it's just like picking the right Lego® pieces so we can build the desired Lego®.

Factor #2

Low Grade Inflammation.

Just as hyperinsulinemia and insulin resistance are common factors in all metabolic disorders, inflammation is also found to be at the root cause of all chronic diseases.

The role of inflammation in chronic disease is very complex and it deserves a book of its own. However, I will try my best to keep it as simple and as practical as possible, just to get a snapshot of all the elements that are involved in disease induced by food and lifestyle.

Just as insulin in itself is not bad, inflammation in and of itself is not a bad thing. In fact, it is the normal response of our body to injuries.

We can detect two types of inflammation: acute, and chronic or low-grade (also known as chronic global inflammation).

An example of acute inflammation would be a paper cut when the area that's injured gets red, warm, swollen and painful. These are all classic signs and symptoms of acute inflammation and are a normal response to an injury, which, in fact, initiates the healing process.

Silent/chronic or low-grade inflammation, on the other hand, is the type that's present in chronic degenerative diseases. This type of inflammation is not accompanied by the classical symptoms of acute inflammation, pain, redness, swelling and heat. Low grade inflammation is below the threshold of pain, so it often goes undetected for many years before it makes itself noticed through clinical manifestations. Hence, the name, silent inflammation. It slowly corrodes the organism at a cellular level. Not knowing about it doesn't mean it isn't happening.

I like to think of acute inflammation as the pressure cooker, which starts to whistle when the temperature is too high. It gives you a loud and clear warning, so you know there is danger and you reduce the heat. Silent inflammation is like a slow cooker: the heat is so low that you have to leave it on for hours in order to cook the food. It goes slow, silent, and almost undetected. You don't know it's cooking, or that it's ready until many hours later when you begin to smell the cooked food the same way you would with a pressure cooker.

Diagram #5: Acute & Silent Inflammation

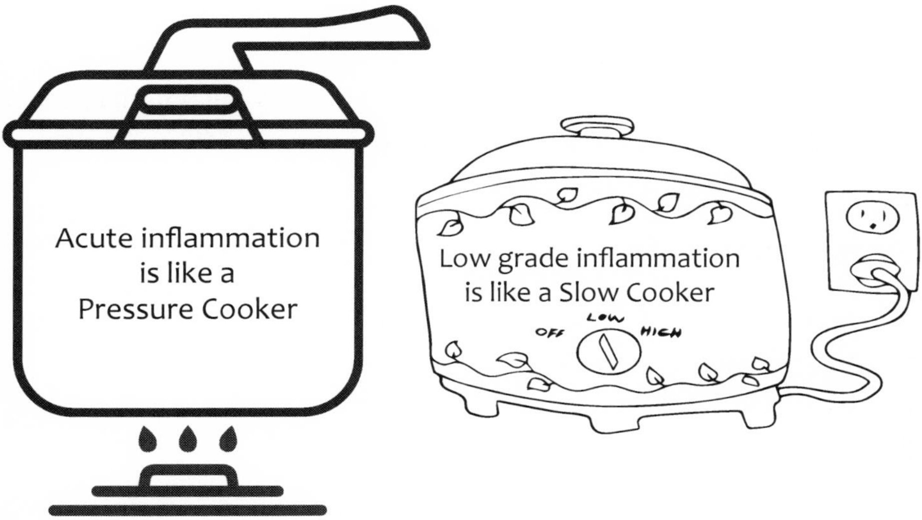

Acute inflammation is like a Pressure Cooker

Low grade inflammation is like a Slow Cooker

OFF LOW HIGH

That's how silent inflammation affects your organs: slowly, without any warning signs, or through very subtle ones, which usually go unnoticed or are attributed to the aging process. *"I must be getting older, that's why I get more headaches or I'm stiff in the morning,"* you might say. Then, as time passes, you begin to accumulate diagnoses: you have asthma, allergies, chronic headaches or migraines, joint pain, diabetes, obesity, cancer, auto-immune diseases, Alzheimer's disease, etc.

You may ask, *"How do I know I have silent inflammation if it doesn't give warning signs, like the acute one does?"*

Inflammation is mediated by a class of hormones known as eicosanoids. The eicosanoids are the ones that are responsible for the pain. We have drugs that actually help us control inflammation by altering the level of eicosanoids in our blood. Whether it's a non-steroidal, anti-inflammatory drug such as aspirin or ibuprofen, or it's a steroidal type of drug such as prednisone or cortisone, the drugs work by affecting the levels of the pro-inflammatory eicosanoids. So, if we reduce the levels of pro-inflammatory eicosanoids, we control pain and we control inflammation. Wonderful! We have the solution: take medication, get rid of inflammation. This can work well, with acute inflammation. If you have a toothache, earache (otitis), headache, back pain, or any other form of acute inflammation, you may take an anti-inflammatory over the counter or prescription drug and that will help rapidly reduce the pain and the inflammation. It's a short-term solution for an acute problem.

However, treating long-term inflammatory processes that involve silent, chronic, low-grade inflammation with anti-inflammatory drugs will result in you suffering from the side effects of these medications, such as immune suppression, osteoporosis, heart problems, and hyperglycemia. Often, the side effects of the drugs can actually be worse than the inflammation itself. It's not uncommon to see people taking one drug to manage a problem and three more to manage the side effects caused by the initial drug.

The good news is that the inflammatory and the anti-inflammatory eicosanoids are food derived. Yes, by changing what you eat, you can actually control low grade global inflammation and the conditions associated with it.

First things first, let's define eicosanoids. The medical definition by The Merriam Webster Dictionary is: *"any of a class of compounds (as the prostaglandins, leukotrienes, and thromboxanes) derived from polyunsaturated fatty acids (as arachidonic acid) and involved in cellular activity."*[16]

I know that probably doesn't mean very much to you. Let me explain in human terms what they are, and how food and lifestyle fit into the inflammatory picture.

Eicosanoids are produced in our body from the fats we eat. Up to this point, we've gotten a good understanding about how carbohydrates, as a macronutrient, contribute to metabolic disorders. It is worth mentioning that a diet low in carbohydrates (such as the metabolic reset protocol) is anti-inflammatory as well. Many (not all) studies done on low carb, high fat diets reported a significant reduction in inflammatory markers such as CRP (C reactive protein) and IL-6 (interleukin -6).[21] Now, it is time to see how fat fits into the picture of disease by its pro-inflammatory or anti-inflammatory effects.

We have two classes or series of eicosanoids. One is the anti-inflammatory series and the other one is the pro-inflammatory series. They are responsible for controlling not only inflammation, but also brain, heart and immune system functions. Some examples of eicosanoids include prostaglandins, thromboxanes, leukotrienes, hydroxylated fatty acids, lipoxins and resolvins.

For nomenclature purposes, the two series of eicosanoids are assigned numbers. Those of odd numbers (series 1, 3 and 5, e.g. PG1 and PG3) are the "good" ones, the anti-inflammatory ones; while those of even numbers (series 2 and 4, e.g. PG2, TXA2) are the "bad" ones, the pro-inflammatory ones.

Coming up next, diagram #6 illustrates the two classes of eicosanoids with their precursor's fatty acids.

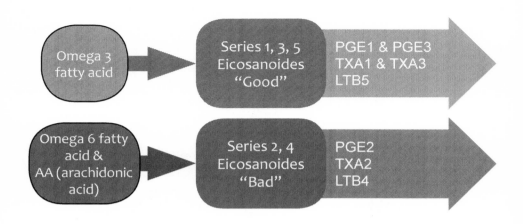

Diagram #6: Eicosanoids classes

I really don't like calling them good or bad, as they are all good when they are in the right ratio. We need the "bad" ones as much as we need the "good" ones. They are the ones that alert us about things not going well and initiate the healing process. The issue comes when there is a gross imbalance between the two, such as too many of the pro-inflammatory versus the anti-inflammatory ones.

This imbalance is mainly caused by our food choices. Let's see why and how.

Omega-6 and omega-3 essential fatty acids are the main ingredients the body uses to make eicosanoids. Another fatty acid that's used primarily for the synthesis of the pro-inflammatory eicosanoids is arachidonic acid (AA). I'll explain more about those fats and the food sources, in the Fat 101 section. Omega-6 and omega-3 fats are essential, meaning we need to acquire them from the diet; our body cannot produce them.

Omega-6 are considered inflammatory fats and omega-3 are the anti-inflammatory ones. What's really important, however, is the ratio of these two fats in the body. Our modern diets provide us with ample amounts of omega-6 fats, but not enough omega-3. That sets the foundation for a rather inflammatory dietary environment with a ratio of omega-6 to omega-3 as high as 20:1, where an ideal ratio should land around 3:1. Diagram #7 illustrates it well.

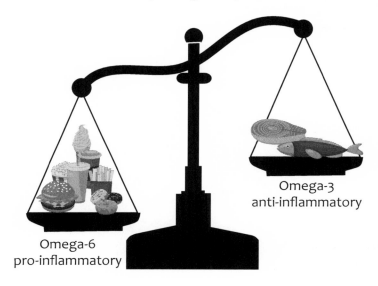

Diagram #7: Omega-6 : Omega-3 ratio

Omega-6 fats are the primary substrate for the production of inflammatory eicosanoids, while omega-3 are for the production of anti-inflammatory ones. The more omega-6 fats we eat, the more of the pro-inflammatory eicosanoids we'll produce.

The main source of omega-6 fats in our diet today are the refined vegetable oils (corn, soybean, sunflower, safflower) and margarines. These are present in all processed, packaged foods (breads, cookies, chips, and all baked goods). Most restaurants use these oils for cooking. On the other hand, the anti-inflammatory omega-3 fats are primarily of marine origin, found in fatty, cold-water fish. Some examples are sardines, mackerel, anchovy, salmon, and trout. From plant sources we have flax seeds, hemp and chia seeds.

This is good and bad news at the same time. It means if you eat too many of the 6s and not enough of the 3s, you promote inflammation. The opposite is also true.

Food becomes like a double-edged sword: one side heals and the other side kills. The choice is yours. You chose what you eat three, or even more, times a day. Food is the most powerful "drug" you will ever have access to; a drug that has the power to heal or to kill. You determine which way it goes. I hope this is good news and it gets you empowered to take action like never before.

I will say this again: "knowledge is power." The real power comes from taking action! By reading this book you are already one step ahead; now you are building up your knowledge, so you can take action from a place of clarity and confidence.

There is more to the omega-6 fats and their conversion into eicosanoids story. Depending on what hormones are present in the blood when we metabolize them, we can change the course of eicosanoid synthesis from pro-inflammatory to anti-inflammatory ones. The diagram below will help you visualize this so it seems less overwhelming.[15]

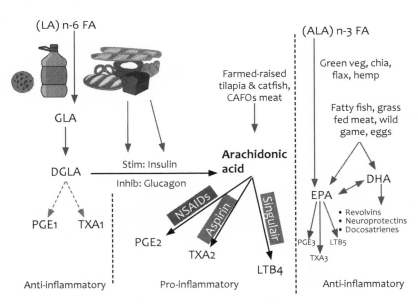

Diagram #8: Eicosanoids synthesis 101

Omega-6 (linoleic acid-LA) is converted to gamma linoleic acid (GLA), which in turn is converted to dihomo gamma linoleic acid (DGLA). Now, DGLA is the key element in here. This can go either the inflammatory route by being converted into arachidonic acid (AA), the inflammatory one, or by being converted into anti-inflammatory eicosanoids (PGE1, TXA1).

What flips the switch? The presence of the insulin![14]

Insulin is a pro-inflammatory hormone. In the presence of insulin, DGLA converts to AA. Insulin activates the enzyme that controls this conversion (delta 5 destauraze enzyme). In the absence of insulin and the presence of glucagon, the same enzyme is suppressed and DGLA is converted into anti-inflammatory eicosanoids.

Thus, the macronutrient composition of your meal is very important, not only when it comes to metabolic health, but to inflammation as well. Food is medicine!

Isn't this incredibly good news? You choose what you eat and you can heal with food! By understanding how the food you eat can drive or stop chronic inflammation, you can virtually reverse any chronic degenerative condition that has inflammation at its root cause.

What are some of those?

- Asthma, allergies, arthritis, joint pain, ulcerative colitis and other inflammatory bowel disease, autoimmune diseases, metabolic syndrome and obesity, various cancers, Alzheimer's disease, diabetes, cardiovascular disease, gum disease, migraine headaches, and other pain.

As you can see they are almost the same ones as those induced by hyperinsulinemia and IR. I am not surprised, as they are all induced by the modern food and lifestyle.

Can you see how we now have more and more Lego® pieces that we know how to use to create the Lego® structure of a *"healthy, happy, vibrant life?"*

At a Glance: Macronutrients and Inflammation

Carbohydrates. Overconsumption of insulinogenic carbohydrates drives hyperinsulinemia, insulin resistance and all associated metabolic disorders. Keeping insulin low not only helps reverse metabolic disorders, but has an indirect anti-inflammatory effect too.
What should you do about it?
  ☐ Dial down foods high in insulinogenic carbs.

Fats. The balance of omega-6 and -3 fatty acids sets the foundation for low-grade inflammation by promoting the production of inflammatory eicosanoids.
What should you do about it?
  ☐ Ditch vegetable oils, margarines and all processed foods made with them; and
  ☐ Dial up omega –3 rich fatty fish.

Proteins stimulate glucagon, which promotes an anti-inflammatory environment by supporting the production of anti-inflammatory eicosanoids.
What should you do about it?
  ☐ Eat your protein with good fat and non-insulinogenic carbs.

Now that we have a good understanding of how inflammation can be controlled by the food we eat, let's see how we can measure low grade inflammation.

Thanks to advancements in modern medicine today, we have ways to test for low grade inflammation that may be going on silently in the body. It's important to know as early as possible so we can intervene with diet and lifestyle to change the outcome.

One laboratory test commonly used to measure inflammation is called CRP or **C reactive protein**. This is a protein produced in the liver in response to any inflammatory process in the body—acute or chronic, it doesn't differentiate between these two. In other words, it's nonspecific. It's elevated by any abnormal condition—anything from the common cold to cancer.

A more specific test that is usually ordered to measure risk for cardiovascular disease is the highly sensitive CRP (hsCRP). Elevation of hsCRP is a good indicator of chronic inflammation that plays a major role in atherosclerosis. [12]

The American Heart Association and U.S. Centers for Disease Control and Prevention have defined risk groups based on hsCRP levels, as follows:

- Low risk: less than 1.0 mg/L
- Average risk: 1.0 to 3.0 mg/L
- High risk: above 3.0 mg/L

Homocysteine is another test worth mentioning. When this amino acid (homocysteine) is found elevated in the blood, it's associated with increased cardiovascular risk.

Low levels of vitamins B6, B12, folate, renal disease, as well as a genetic defect, are possible causes for the elevation of homocysteine.

If you have elevated homocysteine levels it may be a good idea to have a genetic test for the SNIP in the MTHFR gene. This gene provides instructions for making an enzyme called methylenetetrahydrofolate reductase, which is involved in the conversion of a molecule called 10-methylenetetrahydrofolate to a molecule called 5-methyltetrahydrofolate. If this reaction is impaired, then the conversion of homocysteine to another amino acid, methionine, is affected and homocysteine levels build up in the blood. This can be corrected by proper supplementation with a methylated form of folic acid. Testing for the genetic defect is highly recommended. [13]

When it comes to values, most laboratories report homocysteine levels as:

- Normal: 4 - 15 micromoles/liter (μmol/L)

- High: > 15

- Optimal: below 10 to 12

There are other blood tests I recommend doing for early detection of inflammatory and metabolic disorders. You will find those in the section *"now that you know, what do you do."*, on page 201.

I'd like to add one more factor that actually complicates things even more when it comes to understanding inflammation, obesity, and metabolic disorders.

The adipose tissue is now considered to be an endocrine organ. It secretes a class of humoral factors (adipokines) and in obese individuals (primarily the visceral fat, the one that accumulates inside the abdominal cavity) it shifts to producing inflammatory cytokines (another class of chemicals/proteins that modulate inflammation). Just like the eicosanoids, the cytokines are also inflammatory and anti-inflammatory. The fat-released cytokines seem to also be involved in the low grade systemic inflammation seen in metabolic syndrome and arterial disease.[15]

What does this mean? Inflammation can be driven externally by the foods we eat and internally by the chemicals released by the adipose tissue. Thus, by making diet and lifestyle changes that support weight loss, we also reduce inflammation driven by the fat tissue itself.

To this day there is a question that doesn't have a clear answer: what comes first, inflammation or obesity? I don't believe there is a need to wait for the answer. You can start to take action now and change the outcome of your life by getting rid of both of them.

Awareness Exercise:

Begin by reading the food labels of everything you purchase, should it come with one.

First, read the ingredients. Does it have oil? What kind? Does it have sugar? When is it listed: first, second, etc.? The ingredients are listed on a package starting with the one that weighs the most and ending with the one that weighs the least. Be mindful, sugar comes under many names (more about this in Carbohydrates 101).

Preferably, you want to buy foods that are not made with vegetable oils and are low in insulinogenic carbohydrates.

If you like to keep track of your macros, you may look at the nutrition facts and see how much fat it has per serving, then how much is listed as omega-6 and omega-3. Choose products that have lower omega-6 and higher omega-3.

Second, look up the total grams of carbohydrates. Subtract the fiber and you'll be left with the insulinogenic carbs (also known as net carbs). The higher the number for the fiber in rapport with the number for the total carbohydrates, the better.

Third, check out the protein content. Keep in mind that, although protein is good for you, too much of a good thing can turn bad.

More about how to use food labels to your advantage will come in the Now That You Know, What Do You Do! section of the book. The purpose of this exercise is to get you used to reading the labels and to raise your awareness about what you're eating.

Factor #3

Gut integrity, Gut Function and the Microbiome.

"All diseases begin in the gut." - Hippocrates

In this section, we are going to look at gut integrity and function and at how the gut microbiome contribute to disease in the body and how food fits into this picture.

It will seem like we're going to shift gears a little bit, but, in the end, you'll see that the dietary and lifestyle changes that we already covered in the insulin and inflammation section greatly overlap with those that are needed to restore gut integrity and function.

This is a topic I'm very passionate about. My entrance into the low carb, high fat world was through the gut restore protocol, called GAPS. The information I'm about to share with you profoundly changed my health and the way I practice nutrition.

I had the privilege to train with one of the pioneers in the field of gut health: Dr. Natasha Campbell McBride. What I'm about to share with you here barely scratches the surface of the depth of gut health and all its implications. For a complete and thorough explanation of this topic I highly recommend reading the book *Gut and Psychology Syndrome: Natural Treatment for Autism, Dyspraxia, A.D.D., Dyslexia, A.D.H.D., Depression, Schizophrenia.*

Now, to my condensed explanation on the importance of healing the gut before we attempt anything else.

When I first started my nutrition studies, back in 2003, I used to think this:

"You Are What You Eat."

Now, more than a decade later, after extensive studies, personal implementation and working with hundreds of individuals, I believe that:

"You Are What You Eat, Absorb and Store."

It's very important that we eat real, fresh food. That's one reason why I started this book by defining food. Secondly, even if we eat the best food possible, if the gut is not healthy, we are not going to absorb the nutrients our body needs. If the nutrients from food are not absorbed then, sooner or later, we develop nutritional deficiencies, which can translate into diseases in different organs or systems of the body, usually the ones that are constitutionally/genetically weaker. In my case, the weaker system was the gut.

Our gut is the root of our health. Everything begins in the gut.

Our digestive tract is not only there to assure we get nourishment, but it's the host of a mass of microbes—mainly found in the large intestine.

I like to think of the human body as a mighty, beautiful fruit tree. The root of this tree is the gut. The digestive system and the microorganisms that inhabit our gut (gut flora or the microbiome) are the soil in which our gut plants its roots. Healthy soil (gut microflora) supports the growth of strong roots (a healthy, well-functioning gut), which leads to a healthy tree with beautiful green leaves and lots of fruit. You can think of the fruit as the health and the ability to do so many wonderful things in life. The food we eat and the lifestyle we have are the equivalent of the water and the sun a tree needs to get, in order to grow and to bear fruits, while having its roots planted firmly in rich nourishing soil. See Diagram #9.

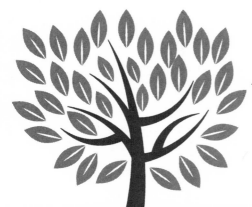

The tree represents a healthy human

The soil represents a balanced gut flora

The roots represent a healthy functioning gut

Diagram #9: Tree of human healthy

To understand how our gut functions and the importance of gut lining integrity and nutrient absorption we need to talk about gut flora first. Microorganisms inhabit our gut and the rest of our body. It has been stipulated that 90% of our genetic material is made of microbes. For every human cell there are 10 micro-organism cells. We are a mass of microbes with a human face. The health of those microbes, the balance between the "good" and the "bad" ones, is what sets the stage of gut health and human health. They serve so many roles in human health that I don't think we could live without them. From nutrient absorption, to energy generation and immune system maturation and function, microbiota play a crucial role in it all.[45]

As you probably know by now, I always look back to how our ancestors lived and try to learn from them. They lived in close contact with the earth and its microorganisms; it was a permanent exchange of microbes between us and our environment. Today, we live in an almost sterile environment. We use anti-microbial soaps and wipes, and everything else we can to keep microbes away. That is not all that good for us.

Before we get into the effects on our health caused by an imbalanced gut flora, let's see first what healthy gut flora looks like and what it does for us.

Human gut flora is comprised of three classes of microbes:

- essential microorganisms (or probiotics);

- opportunistic (or pathogenic); and

- transitional.

Rather than thinking some are bad and some are good, think of the balance between the three classes as being the crucial factor. When the essential flora is present in the greatest number, then the other two are kept under control and they serve their role in our gut ecology and health.

Have you noticed that this is the same when it comes to insulin and inflamma-tion? Too much insulin is the problem, too many pro-inflammatory eicosanoids are the problem, too many of the pathogenic microbes are the problem. It's the yin and yang of life. We can't say that night is bad because it's dark; we need the night to rest and reset so we can enjoy the day. It would be bad if there would be no more daylight; that would be a state of imbalance.

Same goes when it comes to the good and bad microbes that live in symbiosis with us. When the bad ones outnumber the good ones, then things start to go sour.

The many roles gut flora plays in human health
• *Protection from invaders*
• *Appropriate digestion and absorption*
• *Vitamin production*
• *Detoxification*
• *Immune system modulation*
• *Maintaining the health and integrity of the gut*
All those functions, as you can imagine, are very important for us.

Next, I will explain the health and integrity of the gut lining, as this is relevant to understanding gut health and how it affects the rest of our body.

Gut Structure 101.

The intestinal cells are called enterocytes and they are the major player in digestion and absorption of nutrients. Although the intestines are pipe-like looking, the absorptive surface of the small intestine is not flat, it looks like fingers (protrusions). Those finger-like protrusions are called villi and point towards the lumen of the intestine. The villi are covered with a single layer of cells—the enterocytes—and that's where the absorption and final digestion of the nutrients coming from food takes place.

Each enterocyte is covered with hair-like filaments (microvilli, also known as the brush border). Those filaments are covered with enzymes (brush border enzymes). The enterocytes are extremely active cells, and they have a very short life span of approximately 48-72 hours. Once they live their short life's purpose of helping us digest and absorb nutrients, they shed off from the tip of the finger-like villi and die. Then, new ones are born from the base of the finger-like villi.

lumen of small intestine

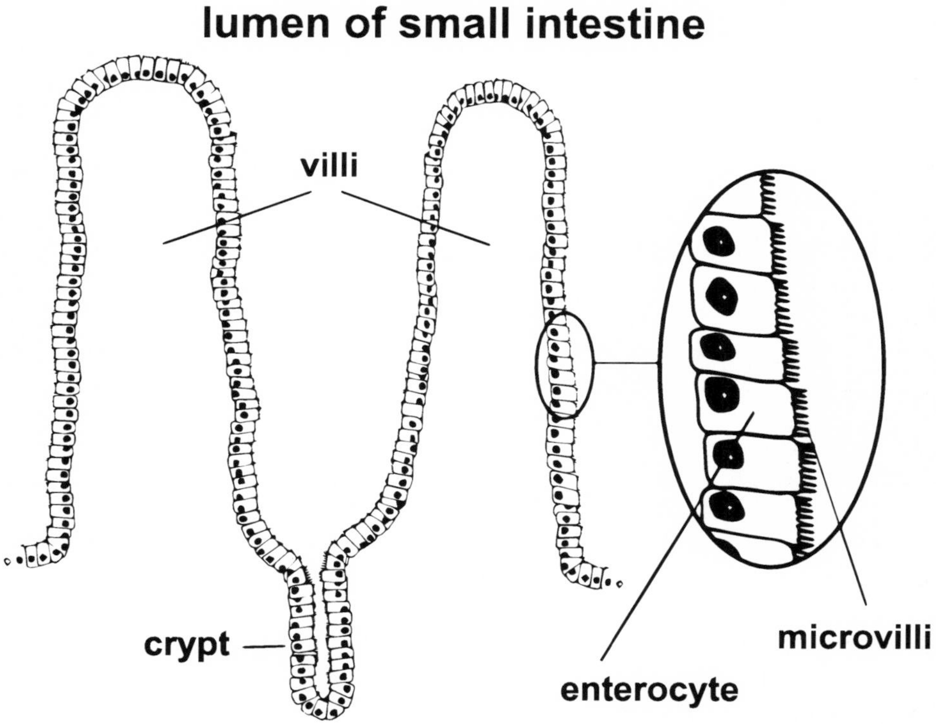

Diagram #10: Gut structure

The enterocytes are kept very tight together by a protein-like glue, which makes the gut lining a semi-permeable membrane. In other words, it allows the absorption of nutrients, but only of a particular size; no undigested food molecules can pass in between them. We can say that the enterocytes form an invisible gut barrier. The invisible link between the enterocytes is called the "tight junctions."

The gut barrier is in many ways very similar to the blood brain barrier, which is also semi-permeable and only allows passage to the brain of certain sized molecules that are safe for the master organ: the brain. This has relevance later when we'll talk about ketones as a brain fuel.

Think of a healthy gut lining as a very dense sieve, or a cheese cloth, which is perfect for straining the finest particles out. When you use it, only the liquid and the finest size particles pass through. Similarly, a healthy gut only allows the absorption of fully digested nutrients of "the approved" size.

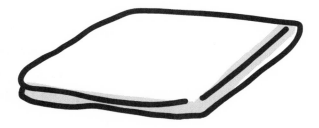

Cheese cloth

Now, why all this explanation? Because the structure and the function of the enterocytes and their finger-like filaments covered in enzymes (the brush border enzymes) are orchestrated by the well-balanced gut flora. The birth, maturation and function of the enterocytes, the brush border enzyme secretion, the final digestion and absorption of nutrients, and the strength of the tight junctions are all directly controlled by the beneficial microorganisms. If the gut flora is compromised, it initiates a domino effect and everything, from the integrity of the gut lining to the ability to produce enzymes, digest and absorb nutrients, gets compromised.

"All diseases begin in the gut," Hippocrates said over 2000 years ago, and he was correct.

Let's see what damages the gut flora and how that affects us. The list is rather long, but I think it is worth mentioning it here, as most of these are modifiable factors:

- Antibiotics, steroid drugs, contraceptive pills, pollution, radiation, alcohol, toxic chemicals, dental work, diseases, chlorine, acute and prolonged stress, and poor diet.

Our modern lifestyle is a big threat to our gut flora balance. When gut flora gets out of balance, with less of the beneficial microorganisms and more of the pathogenic ones, our health slowly begins to deteriorate from the roots up. If these roots get weak (gut and digestive function), soon the trunk (your body) will too.

Keep in mind, this doesn't happen overnight. Just as we discussed with hyperinsulinemia, insulin resistance and low grade inflammation, things happen slowly and over a long period of time before they surface as disease. Again, ignorance is not bliss; not knowing doesn't mean it doesn't happen.

So, when the gut flora is abnormal, the gut deteriorates; its structure and function are affected. Pathogens and toxins coming from food, water and the environment damage the enterocytes and weaken the tight junctions. Many pathogenic microbes in the abnormal gut flora also produce toxins which dissolve that glue-like protein and open the tight junctions as well. So, the gut becomes porous and leaky, allowing "banned" substances to go through and enter the bloodstream.

Remember how we said the gut is like a cheese cloth? Now, it becomes like a pasta strainer with big holes, and it loses the barrier function. Instead of being a semi-permeable membrane, it becomes a freeway, allowing the passage of pretty much anything from the lumen of the intestine into the bloodstream.

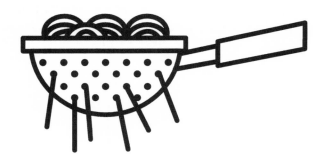

Pasta strainer

That is not good!

The immune system becomes bombarded with foreign substances (pathogens, toxins and partially digested foods) and it initiates an attack against them. Inflammatory processes starting from the gut begin to spread into the whole body.

One of the foreign substances that the immune system begins to fight against are partially digested foods.

When the gut is leaky, large molecules of food that are only partially digested pass into the bloodstream, but in this form, they are not recognized as food; hence, the immune system starts to fight against the food you eat. It responds with low grade inflammation, food sensitivities and intolerances.

Food may be organic, whole and fresh, but if it gets in the bloodstream in a form your immune system doesn't recognize as safe, it will trigger an inflammatory response against it. In this case, there is nothing wrong with the food; it is the damaged gut lining, the state of leaky gut, or gut hyper permeability, which is the cause of this phenomenon.

Food allergies and intolerances can cause many symptoms in the body, from headaches to abnormal behavior to arthritis. The reaction can show itself immediately, in a few hours or in a few days. As these reactions overlap with each other; it is nearly impossible for you to figure out what you are reacting to.

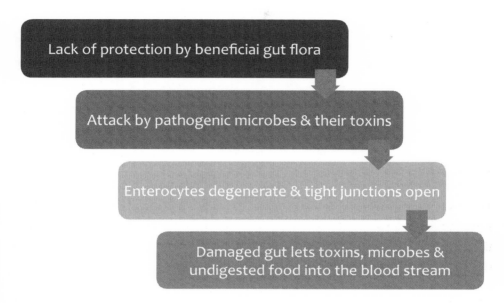

Diagram #11: Leaky Gut 101

The solution is not to eliminate the foods that cause a reaction. The solution is to support the gut to produce new healthy enterocytes, to close the tight junctions between them, and to restore its semi-permeable barrier-like function. Once the gut lining heals, food intolerances and sensitivities will disappear. That's not to say that eliminating foods that trigger inflammation will not provide temporary relief. It will. As the elimination is in place, the focus should be on healing the gut and restoring gut flora balance. It's a double fold approach.

There are several theories of how autoimmunity develops. Here I will describe one possibility, which shows that autoimmunity has its deep, primordial roots in the gut.

The immune system is malnourished due to poor nutrient absorption, which has been going on for a long time. As gut function continues to deteriorate, the immune system is bombarded with many toxins, pathogens and partially digested foods coming from the leaky gut. The immune system becomes overwhelmed and overworked. It reaches a breaking point where it can no longer distinguish safe and self from dangerous and foreign. When this happens, it starts fighting against the body's own tissues, as they no longer seem safe. It may fight against thyroid cells and cause autoimmune thyroiditis (Hashimoto's), or against connective tissue and cause Rheumatoid Arthritis, or against the myelin sheath that covers the nerves and cause Multiple Sclerosis. Autoimmune attacks on the body add more damage on top of what the toxins and pathogenic microbes are already doing.

In reality, things are much more complicated than I described them here, but this is for you to see how, although you may suffer from a disease that affects an organ of the body that has nothing to do with the gut, by "fixing" the gut you can "fix" the whole body. In other words, Hypocrites was correct over 2000 years ago when he said: *"All diseases begin in the gut."* How did he know it then? Why did it take us more than 2000 years to figure it out? I'm not sure, but I'm glad we know, and I'm glad that you and I can take action to change the state of our health. We can build the Lego® of a *"healthy, happy, vibrant life."*

Now that you have a better understanding of the gut, its structure and function as well as the crucial role played by gut microbes in gut integrity, nutrient absorption and immune function, you probably want to know what to do to keep your gut healthy or to restore its function.

At the beginning of this chapter, I mentioned that the nutritional intervention for repairing the gut is actually very similar to the one needed to reverse hyperinsulinemia, IR and global low-grade inflammation: it's about the carbohydrates again. This is good news, because when you make this change in your diet and lifestyle you have a good chance in addressing all three disease-causing factors: insulin resistance, inflammation, and leaky gut.

Let's see what's needed to repair the gut, restore digestion, absorb nutrients and restore immune function and its balance:

- First, eat whole foods. Absolutely no processed, industrialized, chemicalized food-like substances should be consumed;

- Second, eliminate foods that are difficult to digest and absorb by a gut that's leaky, overpopulated by bad microbes, and that lacks intestinal digestive enzymes (brush border enzymes). Those are carbohydrate containing foods;

- Third, nourish the gut with healing foods that supply the building blocks to forming new and healthy enterocytes; and

- Finally, re-inoculate the gut with friendly microorganisms to help re-establish gut flora balance.

In this section, I will focus only on understanding carbohydrate elimination. The other steps will be discussed in great detail in the "Gut Reset Protocol."

Carbohydrates and the Gut.

All carbohydrates are made of small molecules called monosaccharides (mono=single, saccharide=sugar). These are glucose, fructose, and galactose. Some foods contain only monosaccharides, such as honey or ripe fruits, which contain glucose and fructose.

Other foods contain disaccharides (di=two), or two molecules of monosaccharides bound together, such as sucrose, lactose, maltose.

- Sucrose is glucose-fructose (e.g. table sugar).

- Lactose is glucose-galactose (e.g. milk).

- Maltose is glucose-glucose (e.g. from starch digestion).

Some foods also contain polysaccharides (poly=many). Starch, for example, is a polysaccharide. It's a very long chain with many branches of glucose molecules bound together.

Here's the key element: we absorb into the bloodstream only monosaccharides.

Foods that contain complex sugars (disaccharides and polysaccharides) require more pre-absorptive digestion by the salivary and pancreatic enzymes (mainly amylase), while the final steps of separating the disaccharides into monosaccharides are done by the brush border enzymes.

When the gut lining is compromised, or when the enterocytes are unhealthy and unable to produce adequate amounts of those enzymes, double-sugars—like sucrose (in sugar), lactose (in milk), or maltose (from partial digestion of starch)—can't be split into mono-sugars; hence, they can't be absorbed from the small intestine into the bloodstream.

When this happens, those sugars pass into the large intestine and become food for the pathogenic microbes, and further exacerbate the imbalance in the gut flora.

By eliminating foods that are abundant in those sugars, we accomplish two major goals:

- One is to allow time for the gut wall to turn over and produce new and healthy enterocytes (new ones are born every 72 hours), properly equipped with brush border enzymes. Give them time to rest and repair; and

- Second is to stop feeding the pathogenic gut flora with those double or poly-sugars.

This elimination diet is based on the Specific Carbohydrate Diet and it's also one of the pillars of the GAPS protocol developed by Dr. Natasha Campbell McBride.

In Practical Terms:

For a period of time, you will eliminate from your diet foods that are a rich source of complex sugars. These include:

☐ all starch containing foods (grains, legumes, starchy vegetables)

☐ milk

☐ sugar

What carbohydrate containing foods will you be able to eat?

☐ fruits (fully ripe and in season)

☐ honey

☐ homemade yogurt, kefir

☐ sour cream

☐ nuts, seeds

☐ non-starch containing vegetables (these usually grow above the ground from spring to fall; they come with many rainbow-like colors and have high water content).

For the complete list of gut healing foods, see the Gut Reset Protocol.

Protein and the Gut

Proteins are similar in the digestion process to carbohydrates. They are made of many small units called amino acids bound together (long chains of amino acids are called peptides). Just as we can only absorb carbohydrates as single sugars, we can only absorb protein as single amino acids.

Upon ingestion, proteins are "chopped" into peptides, smaller chains of amino acids. Peptides go from two (dipeptides) to many (polypeptides). This first pre-absorptive step, which prepares proteins for absorption, is done in the stomach by the hydrochloric acid and pepsin (a gastric enzyme), then in the small intestine by pancreatic enzymes (trypsin, chymotrypsin and carboxypeptidase). [19]

The final step, when the dipeptides or polypeptides reach the stage of passing through the brush border of the enterocytes into the bloodstream, is when the brush border enzymes split them into single amino acids.

When the gut integrity is compromised (leaky gut), the proteins are absorbed into the bloodstream partially digested as di- or polypeptides, not as single amino acids. This triggers an immune response, as they are not recognized as food or safe.

Gluten from grains and casein from milk are two proteins that we know are absorbed as peptides. They cause severe inflammatory responses with multiple clinical manifestations (from mood, to gut, to skin, to joints, to hormones, all can be affected by these two proteins). There are other such proteins that modern nutritional science is studying and will eventually confirm their contribution to disease processes in the human body.

While it's safe to eliminate carbohydrates from the diet, as they are not essential, proteins are a whole other story. They are essential for health and survival. We know that of the 20 amino acids found in our body, 9 are essential and we need to acquire them from diet, as the body can't produce them.

We'll talk about protein and how much is too much in the Protein 101 chapter. For now, let's see how to use protein to heal the gut so we can properly absorb the nutrients and reverse other disease processes.

The most important part when it comes to protein is to choose the easier to digest and absorb forms. Those are of animal origin (eggs, fish, meat). If you have no egg allergy, eggs are a very easy to absorb protein and are packed with so many other power nutrients. If we use common sense, we know eggs have everything that is needed to bring to life a new being (in this case it would be a chicken, duck, or goose), so they must be packed with life giving and life sustaining nutrients.

The way we cook proteins impacts their digestibility:

- Boiling, stewing, poaching, or slow cooking meat is much easier to digest than fried, grilled or roasted meat.

With that being said, the most gut healing food is meat and bone stock. It's a great source of amino acids that are vital for maintaining a healthy gut and immune system.

Collagen is a structural protein made of 2 non-essential amino acids: glycine and proline. It is found abundantly in meat and bone stock. You get a good supply of those amino acids when you eat/drink a gel-like stock.

Gelatin, a fantastic source of collagen, was valued for its medicinal benefits for thousands of years and was long considered a panacea for everything from skin and joint disorders to digestive distress to heart ailments to the common cold. [34]

Did you know that chicken stock is also called "Jewish Penicillin"? Somehow, they figured out that chicken stock was healing before modern science did. Never underestimate the power of traditional wisdom!

Kitchen Tips:

To make gelatin or a stock that's gel-like when refrigerated, you need to use bones with many joints, such as pork feet or chicken, duck, goose feet or oxtails.

Choose, as your main source of nourishing foods, animal protein and use gentler methods of cooking, such as simmering in a soup, slow cooking in a stew with non-starchy vegetables, poaching, steaming or baking.

Fat and the Gut.

Fat behaves very differently than carbohydrates and protein when it comes to digestion. If you remember from our previous chapter, fat also behaves differently when it comes to its interaction with the hormones that regulate energy metabolism (insulin and glucagon).

Fat stays neutral!

Fat is our best macronutrient friend, yet, we have demonized it for so long that now everybody is afraid of it. Hence, I say let's *Make Peace With Fat!*

As far as we know, the enterocytes don't have to do much work when it comes to fat absorption. The big work is done by the liver in producing bile, and the gallbladder by storing it and releasing it at the right time in the digestive process. Bile prepares the fat by emulsifying it and preparing it for the action of the pancreatic enzymes (lipase).

In people with compromised gut health, however, there is excessive mucus production which interferes with the digestion of all nutrients, including fat. When food particles are coated in mucus, both the bile salt and the digestive enzymes can't properly get to the food to digest it. In this case, when fat is consumed we see fatty stools.

By following the carb elimination diet discussed earlier for a long enough time, the production of mucus normalizes and fat absorption improves. [18]

At this point, we have all the pieces we need to understand how disease and health are influenced by food and lifestyle. In the next section, we're going to dive into understanding macronutrients.

Make Peace With Fat.

Learn to embrace fat!

In "Fats 101," you will understand which fats are bad for you, as some are.

For now, just begin to think, *"Fat is my friend," "I'm ready to make peace with fat."*

How to approach fat?

If you've been following a low-fat diet for a long time, start reintroducing fat into your diet in a slow fashion.

- Increase the amount slowly, so your body has time to adapt to digesting and burning fats again.
- Your body will start to produce and release bile and the enzymes needed to support fat digestion, and the mitochondria will become more proficient at burning fat for fuel.

If you don't have a gallbladder or you find that you have difficulty digesting fats (you may feel nauseous or you may see floating, fatty stool), it's a good idea to add a digestive enzyme that comes with Ox bile to your meals.

- Finally, be patient! As you begin to eliminate the foods high in complex carbohydrates, your gut will restore its function. Soon you'll better digest and absorb all nutrients, including fat.

KNOWLEDGE

PART 3:
MACRONUTRIENTS

So far I've talked about how macronutrients interact with hormones, and how they are absorbed at the intestinal level. We looked at food through the scientist's eye, and not as much at food in a way that you may relate to. Now, it's time to look at food through the chef's eye; to look at what goes on your shopping list and, ultimately, on your plate; and how that relates to healing, energy and performance.

Food, the way nature provides it to us, is a mix of macronutrients and micronutrients.

> Macro=big. Macronutrients come in larger amounts (carbohydrates, proteins and fats). Micro=small. Micronutrients come in minute amounts (vitamins, minerals and trace minerals).

An interesting fact about whole foods is that in nature we can't find a food that's 100% one single isolated macronutrient. The one that comes the closest to being one macronutrient only (carbohydrate) is honey, and even honey has 0.1 g of protein per 1 tablespoon.

You may ask how about olive oil, butter, agave nectar, or whey protein powder? These are single macronutrients, but of course, they are man-made products, not true naturally made foods.

Some foods are higher in one macronutrient than the rest, so we tend to look at them as a "protein" (e.g. eggs, fish, cheese, beef), or a "carbohydrate" (e.g. banana, watermelon, bread, rice, oatmeal, potato, sweet potato), or as "fat" (e.g. avocado, nuts, olives, bacon).

A general rule to help you remember macronutrients in food is:

- carbohydrates are present in all plant foods;

- the only animal food that contains a significant amount of carbohydrates is milk (sugar in milk called lactose);

- fats are found in all foods of plant and animal origin; and

- proteins are also found in all foods of animal or plant origin.

Let's take a look at each macronutrient and the main food source we find it in.

CARBOHYDRATES

3.1 CARBOHYDRATES 101

Not all carbs are created equal! In this section, we are going to look at carbohydrates':

- Energetic value

- Main role in the body

- Food sources

- Insulinogenic and non-insulinogenic carbohydrates

- Net carbohydrates (NC)

Energetic Value of Carbohydrates.

- Carbohydrates, upon digestion and metabolization, provide us with 4 cal/gram.

Main Role in the Body.

Energy:

Carbohydrates are a quickly released form of energy for the body. A fast burning, short lasting fuel. They are absorbed in the form of monosaccharides, with the main one being glucose. Glucose is oxidized aka "burned" to generate energy in the form of ATP, and as byproducts CO_2 and H_2O are also produced. Adenosine triphosphate (ATP) = energy. You may often hear the term "carb burning metabolism"—that's what it refers to: the body is converting glucose into energy.

Structure and function:

> Carbohydrates are part of glycoproteins found in cell membranes and are
> involved in cell-to-cell communication.

There is no essentiality when it comes to the carbohydrates as a main macronutrient. In human terms, that means we do not have to consume carbohydrates in order to survive; our body can produce glucose from non-glucose
compounds such as amino acid and the glycerol bone from fatty acids metabolism, via gluconeogenesis.

Food Sources of Carbohydrates.

We find carbohydrates in all plant foods. They are not all created equal when it
comes to the way we absorb and metabolize them.

Regarding animal foods as a source of carbohydrates, the glycogen stored
in muscle meat is the equivalent of plant starch; however, meat and animal
products don't contain significant amounts of glycogen that can be converted
to glucose. During the stressful event of slaughtering, epinephrine and stress
hormones are released and most of the glycogen is depleted.[52] Milk is the only
animal product that contains an insulinogenic carbohydrate.

Milk, Yogurt, Kefir, Buttermilk, Whey (liquid whey).

The carbohydrate in milk, lactose, is the double-sugar made of glucose and
galactose. As opposed to fruits, legumes, starchy vegetables and grains, milk
being an animal product lacks fiber and that allows for a faster absorption of
glucose in the blood stream. Hence, milk has a significant insulinogenic effect.

> *Due to its insulinogenic effect, milk is not part either of the metabolic or
> the gut rest protocol. Hence you will not see it on any of the shopping
> lists.*

Yogurt and the rest of the fermented dairy products are a different story altogether.

The sugar in fermented dairy products is predigested by the probiotic cultures used to ferment them. They have a lesser insulinogenic effect, are more digestible, and provide us with the beneficial microorganisms that help reestablish gut flora balance and, as a result, heal the gut.

Grains, Legumes and Starchy Vegetables.

Grains are the seeds of grass.

Some examples of grains (gluten and non-gluten containing) are:

- wheat, barley, rye, oats, rice, corn, millet, sorghum, teff, and wild rice.

Pseudo grains (Gluten Free) include:

- amaranth, quinoa, teff, and montinaTM (Indian ricegrass).

Examples of grain products are:

- bread, pasta, oatmeal, breakfast cereals, tortillas and grits, baked goods, pastries, and anything else that's made with flour (cakes, pancakes, waffles, bagels, donuts, etc.).

Legumes are fruits in the form of a pod splitting along both sides, of plants from the family of Leguminosae and include beans, peas, acacia, alfalfa, clover, indigo, lentil**, mesquite, mimosa, and peanut.[46]

Examples of beans are:

- adzuki, black, soybean, fava, anasazi, garbanzo, kidney and lima beans.

*Buckwheat and its flour are used as a gluten free alternative food. Buckwheat is not a grain nor a legume. It is botanically classified as the fruit of a plant that's related to rhubarb and sorrel.

**Lentils come in a variety of colors such as red lentils, green, brown and black lentils, as well as split peas.

Starchy vegetables include foods such as:

- potato and sweet potato, plantains, yuca (from which tapioca flour is made), winter squashes (butternut squash, pumpkin, acorn squash, spaghetti squash), and sweet corn (the one you eat on the cob).

What do grains, legumes and starchy vegetables have in common? They all contain starch.

Starch breaks down in the body into maltose (a double sugar made of two glucose molecules) and is ultimately absorbed as a mono-sugar, glucose which requires insulin for further metabolization.

Two reasons to eliminate starches:

- Reason #1: their insulinogenic effect contributes to insulin resistance and inflammation with all its complications (weight gain, metabolic syndrome, fatty liver, PCOS, diabetes, Alzheimer's disease, etc.).

- Reason #2: they are difficult to digest if gut function and integrity are comprised.

In the next section of the book, Now That You Know, What Do You Do!, you will find the complete shopping list of foods that support reversal of IR and inflammation, as well as, for healing the gut. For a quick look at carbs and their health effect, you can refer to the table *Carbohydrates at A Glance.*

Fruits

Fruits contain the simple sugars (monosaccharides) glucose and fructose, not bound together, which when it comes to digestion, are easily absorbed even when the gut is not completely healthy.

However, fruits are also insulinogenic. So, when it comes to metabolic disease and inflammation; when it comes to losing weight, lowering triglycerides, blood sugar management, reversing insulin resistance or reducing inflammation, fruits don't make it on the shopping list. Or they make it in a small amount, and only very few of them that have higher fiber content and are richer in antioxidants and phytonutrients, such as berries.

On the other hand, if IR and its associated diseases are not a concern for you, and your main priority is your gut integrity and function, then fruits make the shopping list.

That was my case. When I first started on the low carb healing journey, I was in great need to heal my gut. I followed the gut reset protocol, so I continued to eat fruits. However at first I couldn't tolerate hardly any raw foods, due to gas and overall gut distress, so my intake of fruits was somewhat limited by that. Only about 3 years later, I shifted my focus more towards glycemic management and performance. Now, fruits are a very small part of my diet, the very opposite picture compared to what it was when I followed a raw vegan and vegetarian eating style. During those days my diet was extremely high in fruits, both fresh and dry.

I'll explain more on how to approach fruits in the Now That You Know, What Do You Do! section.

A Word about Fructose.

The monosaccharide, fructose, is responsible for the sweet taste of foods. Glucose is less sweet, so if we were to take fructose out of foods, we would probably enjoy them less as they would not be as sweet. Unlike glucose, fructose doesn't require insulin for absorption. It is metabolized by the liver and converted into fat.

We find fructose in higher concentration in fruits, fruit juice, sucrose (sugar), honey, agave nectar and high fructose corn syrup. In fact, all plant foods contain fructose (even kale does). It comes in a lesser amount of course, and it is harder for us to absorb it from whole foods as opposed to their juice.

Since the industrialized era, when fruit juices and fructose corn syrup sweetened beverages, candies, and other processed foods made their way into our diet, we see not only an increase in obesity and type II diabetes, but in the incidence of non-alcoholic fatty liver disease as well. The biggest threat to abdominal obesity and nonalcoholic fatty liver is by far high fructose corn syrup.

Where do you find fructose? In all processed foods, fruit and fruit juices.

So you may ask which one is worse, glucose or fructose? I think they are equally bad for the carbohydrate intolerant person.

Honey.

Honey is an invert sugar formed by an enzyme from nectar gathered by bees. Honey contains fructose and glucose, not bound together. Nevertheless, honey is insulinogenic. If metabolic disorder is your concern, it's best to keep honey out. If you are metabolically healthy, yet you need to reset your gut health, then honey is easy to digest and absorb, plus it has many other nutrients aside from sugar.

Personally, if I need to sweeten something I use honey or dates. In small amounts, I can make it fit within my daily carb balance. In fact, the menu you will find at the end of the book is a good example of this, as honey is part of some recipes.

The good news is, as you go on this low carb-high fat journey, you will crave less and less sweets. Your taste buds will lose the desire for sweet and you'll be happy with the natural sweetness of heavy cream, as an example.

Coconut Sugar is it less insulinogenic than regular sugar?

Most recent to the market, Coconut Sugar is a sugar made from sap, which is the sugary circulating fluid of the coconut plant. As per manufacturers, coconut sugar is 70–79% sucrose, and 3-9% each glucose and fructose, with minor variations. Coconut sugar has slightly less fructose than table sugar, and that may be what makes it better than regular sugar. I personally don't get sold on that argument. Some sources report coconut sugar to have a glycemic Index (GI) of 35, while others say 54.

Just as with all other sugars, coconut sugar elicits an insulin response, so it is no different when it comes to its metabolic effect or when it comes to gut health.

Carbohydrates at a glance.

Food	Examples	Insulino-genic	Gut health
Grains	Wheat, barley, kamut, millet, quinoa, rye, amaranth, oats, etc. and everything made with those	☹	☹
Starchy vegetables	Potatoes, sweet potatoes, yuca, plantain, corn, and winter squashes	☹	☹
Legumes	Dry beans, lentils, split peas, green peas, and soy	☹	☹
Dairy	Milk and store bought yogurt	☹	☹
Fruits and fruit juices	Banana, cherries, apples, oranges, mango, grapes, etc.	☹	☺ as individually tolerated, fully ripe, local and seasonal
Sugar and everything made with sugar, including sugar alcohols	Cane, beet, coconut, turbinado, brown rice syrup, etc.	☹	☹
Honey	Raw, unfiltered	☹ my be able to use in small amount	☺
Non-starchy vege-tables	Leafy greens, cabbage, broccoli, cauliflower, zucchini, mushrooms, bell peppers, etc.	☺	☺ as individually tolerated
Nuts and seeds	Macadamia, pine nuts, walnuts, pecan, hazelnuts, hemp seeds, chia seeds, sunflower seeds, pumpkin seeds, etc.	☺	☺ as individually tolerated

Sugar or Sucrose and everything made with sugar.

Sugar is not on the shopping list either for metabolic or for gut health. Perhaps what's worth mentioning here is that sugar comes under many names so it can be challenging if you eat foods that come in a package/box/bag, etc.

Let's see some of them:

- brown sugar, confectioner's sugar, or powdered sugar;

- raw sugar; sucrose, or table sugar, from sugar canes or sugar beets;

- turbinado sugar is raw sugar that goes through a refining process to remove impurities and most of the molasses;

- molasses, blackstrap molasses and rapadura;

- corn syrups;

- high-fructose corn syrup (HFCS) is a sweetener made from corn-starch;

- dextrose is also known as corn sugar;

- invert sugar;

- lactose, or milk sugar, is made from whey and skim milk for commercial purposes;

- levulose or fructose is known as a fruit sugar, occurs naturally in many fruits;

- date sugar;

- agave nectar;

- brown rice syrup, barley malt, birch sugar and syrup; and

- maple syrup, maple sugar.

Personal reflection on the many names of sugar. *I don't know about you, but for me it's easier to eat whole foods, which don't have food labels, or ingredients lists than to have to read ingredients and to remember all the names under which sugar may hide. But that's, of course, me. Sometimes I still feel like I'm from another planet.*

Sugar Alcohols or Polyols.

Some examples are:

- Sorbitol, mannitol, maltitol, xylitol, and erythritol. They occur naturally in fruits and are produced commercially from such sources as dextrose; and

- Xylitol is a sugar alcohol made from a part of birch trees and corn cobs, or sugar cane bagasse (stalk residue remaining after sugar extraction).

You will find these in sugar free products. They are not calorie free. While sugar has 4 cal/g, sugar alcohols have on average 2 cal/g.

They are considered non-insulinogenic; however, that may not be true and it's a rather controversial topic.

As far as I'm concerned, these fit in the highly-processed food-like substances category. They are not something I personally use or recommend. If you consume them as part of a fruit that naturally contains them (e.g. prunes, a good source of sorbitol), that's different. As isolated compounds, I don't endorse their consumption.

They are fermented by the gut microbes. Their excessive consumption can lead to bloating, abdominal pain, gas and diarrhea. Also, they can change the gut flora balance by supporting the growth of pathogenic microorganisms. According to a study published in Obesity Reviews, high intake of fructose, artificial sweeteners, and sugar alcohols causes the gut bacteria to adapt in a way that interferes with the satiety signals and metabolism. They produce larger amounts of the short chain fatty acids (SCFA) which interfere with satiety signals. We don't feel full and we don't stop eating when we should. [20]

But the biggest problem I see happening when we drop the sugar and replace it with natural or artificial, no calorie sweeteners, is that the taste buds continue to be activated by very sweet stimuli, which doesn't help to get rid of sugar cravings, and it makes it so much more difficult to embrace a lower carbohydrate, higher fat eating style. For as long as we feed the sweet tooth, it will continue to shape our food likes and food choices.

This can be overwhelming. I wanted you to know the many names sugar and sweeteners can show up on processed, packaged foods. You will not have to worry about any of these when you embrace a whole foods eating style, as most whole foods don't come with a food label or a long list of ingredients that are hard to pronounce. That is the beauty of eating clean whole foods!

Green Leafy Vegetables and Non-starchy Vegetables.

As you can see thus far, the bulk of the plant foods we consume today are either providing us sugar (glucose, fructose) or starch (glucose, glucose, glucose), which makes them insulinogenic, inflammatory and not supportive to gut healing.

So you may ask, are there any foods that contain carbohydrates that I can eat?

We have one more class of plant foods we didn't discuss yet: the non-starchy vegetables and the green leafy vegetables. These are our friends when it comes to losing weight, reducing inflammation and keeping our body "clean." Why? These are the "low impact carbs" or non-insulinogenic sources of carbohydrates.

The sugars found in these plants (mostly simple sugars and very small amounts of starch) are well protected inside their cells walls by fiber and diluted by their high natural water content. Another way to look at it is that our gut is not that well equipped to pull out sugar (energy) from those plants. Our gut differs from that of herbivorous animals who are able to extract nutrients and energy from "grass-like" plant foods. See Herbivorous Animals and Plant Digestion, for more insight into this topic.

What makes some of the sugars present in plants more bioavailable to us?

Alterations in fiber, like content and structure. When the fiber is removed or somehow altered, it affects our ability to pull out more sugar and more nutrients from plants.

- Juicing, blending and cooking will make the sugars and the nutrients found in plant foods more bioavailable to us.

Let's take, for example, carrots. Eating raw carrots has a lesser effect on your blood sugar, compared to drinking carrot juice. Carrot juice is a concentrate of sugar, as all the fiber has been removed and the sugars were released from the cell walls into the juice. Also, cooked carrots release more sugar than if you were to eat them raw.

Other examples of vegetables that become more insulinogenic when cooked or when juiced are beets, tomatoes, and onions.

The easiest way for you to identify the vegetables that are least insulinogenic is to think of those that grow above the ground, from spring to fall, come with high water content, and in multiple colors. Some examples of such vegetables are:

- leafy greens (spinach, arugula, dandelion, kale, chard, beet greens, watercress, sorrel, endive, etc.);

- vegetables (cabbage, broccoli, cauliflower, okra, eggplant, mushrooms, tomatoes, cucumbers, bell peppers, celery stalks, asparagus, green beans, zucchini, summer squash); and

- fresh herbs like parsley, cilantro, dill, and basil.

The ones that are behaving a little like starchy vegetables when cooked versus raw include mostly those that grow in the ground, like:

- carrots, beets, celery roots, parsley roots, turnip roots, and onions.

Herbivorous Animals and Plant Digestion

Even herbivorous animals, who have grass as their main source of food, do not digest the fiber themselves. The bacteria that are present in their intestinal tract are responsible for that. They have microorganisms in their stomach(s) which support digestion and absorption of nutrients from grass. They actually turn grass into fat, and that allows those animals to get big and strong (look at the elephant, the rhino, the cow and the bull).

Unlike them, our stomachs are almost sterile and have an extremely low pH, which allows proteins from animal foods to be denatured by the hydrochloric acid, while most of our gut flora are found in our large intestine, where little if any nutrient absorption takes place.

For humans, nutrient absorption happens, primarily, in the small intestine.

What does this mean? It means, plant foods, like grains, legumes, starches, green leafy vegetables, non-starchy vegetables and fruits are actually not very nourishing for the human body. They act more as a cleansing food, as our gut is not properly enzymatically equipped to pull out nutrients from those foods. Many of their nutrients are trapped by the fiber inside the cell walls, and never become fully available for absorption by us.

Take it To the Kitchen

☐ Cooking vegetables makes them release more of their simple sugars, hence it makes them more insulinogenic.

☐ Juicing removes all the fiber, so you are left with just the simple sugars. Those aspects are important particularly if you are trying to manage blood sugar (as a diabetic or pre-diabetic) through diet and lifestyle.

☐ Cooking and juicing improves bioavailability of nutrients from plants.

Have you noticed that all starchy vegetables, grains and legumes require cooking to be consumed by us? In fact, that's one other criteria I like to use when I educate my clients about the different types of carbohydrates.

An easy way to recognize starchy vegetables is: if you have to cook it to eat it, it's most likely an insulinogenic vegetable, which contains starch.

☐ Think of grains and grain products (pasta, rice, bread), legumes such as beans and lentils, or potatoes and sweet potatoes; they all need to be cooked.

The rest of the plant foods are pretty much edible either raw or cooked. That's an indication that they contain very little or no starch.

When consumed raw or juiced, they are more cleansing than when cooked.

Eat your foods whole (juice is not a whole food), and eat a mix of raw and cooked vegetables.

Let's talk about fiber. This is hugely important; not only for gut health, but in relation to how we absorb carbohydrates from plant foods. This is where I will introduce the concept of Net Carbohydrates (NC), another way of referring to the insulinogenic carbohydrates.

Fiber is exclusively found in plant foods.

No fiber is found in animal foods, just as no cholesterol is found in plant foods.

Fiber is a non-digestible carbohydrate, meaning humans do not produce digestive enzymes to break down fiber and to absorb nutrients from it. Fiber reaches the large intestine in an undigested form, where it provides food for the gut flora. Most types of fiber act as a prebiotic, feeding the probiotics present in the large intestine. That's not to say that fiber doesn't feed the pathogenic gut microbes as well, especially when the gut flora is out of balance. Pathogenic microorganisms thrive on sugars, starch and artificial sweeteners, and less on the fiber that comes with whole foods, primarily with greens and non-starchy vegetables.

Although, theoretically, fiber is non-caloric (as it is non-digestible), when it is fermented by the microorganisms in the large intestine, it generates about 2 calories per gram! In other words, the bacteria are turning the fiber into short chain fatty acids. As the Advanced Nutrition and Human Metabolism textbook states, *"No longer can the potential energy in fiber be considered totally unavailable to the human body."* [19]

Fiber doesn't provide us directly with nutrients, yet it is extremely important for keeping our gut flora healthy and supplying energy for the colonocytes (colon cells) so they can perform their job. I like to think of fiber as the compound from food which allows us humans to maintain a symbiotic relationship with the gut microbes.

There are two types of dietary fiber: soluble fiber and insoluble fiber.

- insoluble fibers (cellulose, lignin)
- soluble ones (pectin, gum, mucilages, and some hemicellulose)

When we classify fiber like that it is because we are looking at one of fiber's properties: its water solubility. Whole foods contain a mix of those fibers.

Some foods contain more insoluble fiber than soluble:

- grains and their bran, legumes, root vegetables, and vegetables in the cabbage family

Other contain more soluble than insoluble fiber:

- chia seeds, strawberries, apricots, and asparagus

The two fibers behave differently in the body and have very different health benefits. When eating a whole foods based diet, you will reap the benefits of both.

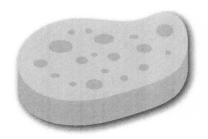

Soluble fiber not only dissolves in water but has the ability to bind to water. It behaves like a dry sponge that absorbs water, toxins and digestive juices. What does this mean to us?

- It turns gel-like and slows down gastric emptying. Food spends more time in the stomach and you feel full for a longer time.
- It also slows down the rate at which glucose is absorbed into the bloodstream, which is a good thing when it comes to blood sugar management and insulin response to food.
- It affects fat and cholesterol absorption by binding to them, and forcing them to be excreted via feces.
- It slows down intestinal transit and interferes to some degree with overall nutrient absorption.

Another characteristic of soluble fiber is its fermentability by the gut microflora. The end result of bacterial fermentation of soluble fibers as well as that of undigested starch that reaches the colon is lactic acid and short chains fatty acids (SCFA).

SCFA supply fuel for the colonocytes and help keep a low pH environment in the colon. Optimal colon pH is ~6-6.5. This may be, in part, responsible for the colon cancer preventative benefits of soluble fiber.

In regards to bowel movements, both soluble and insoluble fiber help increase fecal volume.

Soluble fiber due to its gel formation and water holding capacity delays gastric empting (food spends more time in the stomach which translates in a prolong feeling of fullness), increases transit time (things move slower through the intestines, which is particularly beneficial if you have lose stools).

Insoluble fiber doesn't dissolve in water. It has a lesser water binding capacity and it doesn't turn into a gel-like mass. It actually speeds up transit time, hence, it increases the frequency of bowel movements, a desirable effect if you are constipated and a not so desirable effect if you have diarrhea.

I like to think of insoluble fiber more like a brush that sweeps the inside of our gut. When the gut is ulcerated or inflamed, insoluble fiber causes more harm than good. How would you like to scrub with a brush, even a soft one, on an open wound on your skin? You wouldn't like it, right? When you have gut ulcerations and inflammation, eating foods high in insoluble fiber is like scrubbing an open wound with a brush. It causes more gut irritation, discomfort, and diarrhea.

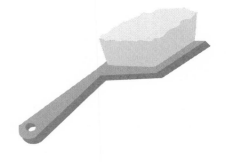

If the gut lining is healthy, eating insoluble fiber is a great way to keep your intestines clean through good frequency of bowel movements and to support detoxification due to bacterial proliferation.

Insoluble fiber is for the most part non-fermentable by the gut microbes, but it promotes the proliferation of the microbes in our colon. This is an extremely valuable property, as the microbes in the colon are responsible for detoxification as well as for an increased fecal volume (bulking action), which is important for proper evacuation, colon health and overall total mind- body health.

Making sure you consume adequate amounts of both types of fiber is crucial to your health maintenance and disease prevention (including colon cancer).

Current recommendations for fiber intake range from 20-40 g/day. It is ok and safe if you go above that. However, when following a low carbohydrate diet that may be difficult to achieve (I mean 40 grams or more of fiber) without adding fiber supplements, such as psyllium husks as an example. I don't have a set number I personally recommend, as each individual has their own unique needs and tolerance according to the state of their gut health.

Personally, when I consume too much fiber, primarily from raw vegetables, I get pain in the large intestine on my left side. I then know I need to back off and stick mostly with cooked vegetables.

It's important to pay attention to how your body responds to the foods you eat. You are the expert on you! You don't need me, or another expert, or a government recommendation to tell you how much of anything you should be eating.

So, what foods are a good source of fiber and are not high in sugar or starch?

I will give you few examples here. There are more, of course, and you'll find them on the shopping list in the next chapter.

Low carb and gut friendly soluble and insoluble fiber rich foods:

- avocado, artichoke, Brussel sprouts, okra, cucumbers, celery, and turnip;

- nuts and seeds (like flax seeds, chia seeds, and hemp seeds); and

- fruits (like berries, figs, and pears).

Keep in mind when adding more "fiber" from vegetables, nuts, seeds or fruits to your diet to do it slowly, in small increments, to allow your gut flora to adapt to it. Doing it this way will decrease the risk of getting gas, bloating, or even diarrhea.

Net Carbohydrates (NC).

Now that you have the complete picture of carbohydrates, from simple sugars to starch to fiber, let's talk about net carbohydrates (NC).

First the formula to calculate net carbohydrates:

Nutrition Facts	
Serving Size	...g
Servings Per Container	
Amount Per Serving	
Calories	Calories from Fat ...
	% Daily Value*
Total Fat ...g	...%
Saturated Fat ...g	...%
Trans Fat ...g	
Cholestrol ...mg	...%
Sodium ...mg	...%
Total Carbohydrate ...g	...%
Dietary Fiber ...g	...%
Sugars ...g	
Protein ...g	
Vitamin A	...%
Vitamin C	...%
Calcium	...%
Iron	...%
*Percent Daily Values are based on a 2,000 calorie diet. Your Daily Values may be higer or lower depending on your calorie needs.	

Total Carbohydrates - Fiber = Net Carbs

Why we use NC and not total carbs? Because, fiber is non-digestible and non-insulinogenic. So, if we extract fiber from the total amount of carbohydrates found in a food, we can estimate the amount of insulinogenic carbohydrates.

Let's take as an example avocado. An avocado of about 9.6 oz. with a pit has 17.1 g of total carbohydrates. This sounds like a lot if we don't take into account how much of it is actually fiber. Let's have a look: 13.5 g of the total carbs in our avocado are actually fiber. That means our avocado has only 3.6 g of absorbable carbohydrates (17.1-13.5=3.6).

Hence, avocados are a low impact food, that doesn't elicit an insulin spike. To learn more about avocadoes refer to the resources section of this book.

The higher the fiber content of the food in relation to to the total carbohydrates, the less insulinogenic the food is.

Alcohol.

Not a food by any stretch of the imagination, but nevertheless it is part of our lives, so it deserves its place in this book. Alcohol provides us with 7 cal/gram.

Many of the commercially available alcoholic beverages are actually high in carbohydrates and are better avoided (e.g. beer, sweet wine, liquors).

There are dry wines that have a lower carb content. Similarly, hard liquor such as vodka, tequila, and whisky have virtually 0 carbs. Those can be part of your life depending on your unique health status and goals.

However, when it comes to alcohol it is not necessarily as much about the carb content, as it is about the ethyl alcohol. The alcohol in hard liquor, very dry wine, or gin doesn't have a direct effect on blood sugar (as it is not converted into glucose), so it doesn't lead to an increase in blood glucose. In fact, quite the contrary, it is well known that alcohol consumption leads to hypoglycemia (low blood sugar), especially for diabetics.

An interesting fact about alcohol is that it is metabolized by the liver as fat and it contributes to fat accumulation in the liver (alcoholic fatty liver). Alcohol actually "hijacks" the liver's ability to produce glucose via gluconeogenesis and it can lead to a drop in blood sugar, especially if consumed on an empty stomach. This is important to keep in mind, especially if you are diabetic.

Now, if you combine the effect of alcohol on the liver with that induced by the consumption of high fructose corn syrup (from all the processed foods and beverages) and a high intake of refined carbohydrates, sodas, and fruit juices, you can see how that can lead to fatty liver, elevation in blood triglycerides, increased abdominal obesity, and consequent metabolic disorders.

My Take on Alcohol.

It depends on your health, health goals and on your relationship with alcohol whether you should eliminate alcohol from your life or not.

If you are not sure what I mean by relationship with alcohol, try three weeks without alcohol.

If you can do it easy, you don't miss it and you are fine with or without it, that means you and alcohol have a healthy relationship. You may enjoy, from time to time, a good glass of dry wine with your dinner. It means alcohol is not your de-stress mechanism at the end of the day.

That's it! I say no more. I'm sure you know exactly what I mean.

If fatty liver and elevated triglycerides are on your list of things you need to "fix," then alcohol is not your friend.

Carbohydrate Intolerance.

It is well recognized that insulin resistance is the driving force behind metabolic syndrome, prediabetes and type II diabetes. The true culprits are actually dietary carbohydrates, as they "demand" insulin from the body.

In other words, in the absence of carbohydrates there is no hyperinsulinemia or insulin resistance. Dr. Voleck, in his book "THE ART AND SCIENCE OF LOW CARBOHYDRATE LIVING," describes *"insulin resistance as carbohydrate intolerance,"* and I must admit I like that way of looking at it. [21]

What does intolerance mean in biology and nutrition? Food intolerance, for instance, refers to difficulty in digesting certain foods.

Now, in the strict sense of the definition, "carbohydrate intolerance" is not characterized by difficulty digesting carbohydrates (from an enzymatic point of view). However, in the metabolic sense, carbohydrate intolerance translates as an inappropriate insulin response to the carbohydrate, which, if not addressed, leads to metabolic disorders.

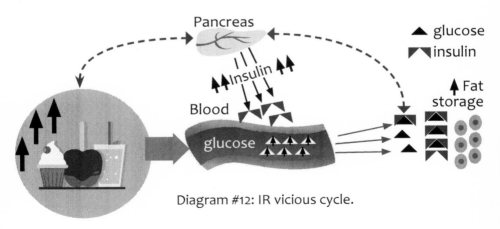

Diagram #12: IR vicious cycle.

Diagram #12 illustrates the concept of IR as a carb intolerance, which leads to excess fat storage (de novo lipogenesis).

What do we do when we have food intolerance?

Let's take as an example gluten or lactose intolerant people. They are advised against consuming foods that contain gluten or lactose. We remove the source of the problem. The problem is not the headache or the diarrhea (that's the physical manifestation, aka. the diagnostic), the problem is the gluten or the lactose and the way the body responds to it.

It's only logical that if we have carbohydrate intolerance, we would follow the same approach: remove the cause of the problem: carbohydrates. That stops the vicious cycle and reverses IR, hyperinsulinemia and all metabolic disorders caused by it. See Diagram #13 below.

When it comes to dietary approaches that eliminate carbohydrates, there are many and they offer a wide range of total carb or NC intake. I like to refer to them as the *"spectrum of low carbohydrate diets."*

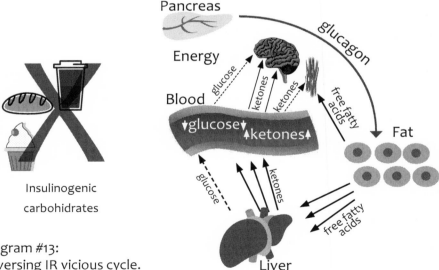

Insulinogenic
carbohidrates

Diagram #13:
Reversing IR vicious cycle.

They range from GAPS, SCD, and Paleo all the way to the Ketogenic diet. They all restrict the amount and types of carbohydrates, and they all aid in the reversal of insulin resistance, inflammation and its associated disorders.

But how do we define a low carb diet? Is there a specific amount of total carbo-hydrates or NC, below which we consider it to be low?

The average American man today consumes about 300 g of carbohydrates a day and the average woman about 225 g/day. Current dietary recommenda-tions are to consume 45% - 60% of your calories as carbohydrates, with a mini-mum of 130 g carbs per day, according to the Institute of Medicine. Clearly this is not considered to be a low carb diet.

> *Personal reflection on current dietary recommendations for carbohy-drate intake.*
>
> *We've been following this advice for the past 50 years or so, and it is pretty obvious that, for the majority of adults in the USA, this doesn't work. We have an epidemic of obesity, diabetes and other metabolic disorders, including cancer and autoimmunity.*

What is a low carbohydrate diet?

If we were to classify it based on grams of carbs consumed per day, it would be:

- Over 150 grams of carbs per day is considered high;

- 100-150 grams of carbs a day is a moderately high carb diet;

- Less than 100 grams a day is getting on the low carbohydrates spec-trum; and

- Less than 50 g/day is considered therapeutic low carb, which is con-ducive to nutritional ketosis and fat burning as primordial fuel. This is the therapeutic low carb we've been talking about in this book.

	Grams of total carbohydrates per day
High	>150
Moderate	100-150
Low	50-100
Therapeutic Nutritional Ketosis	<50

You may ask how about the minimum 130 g of carbs a day recommended by the Institute of Medicine. That's the estimated amount of carbohydrates that the brain requires for its own function. To be more accurate, the brain requires approximately 500-600 cal/day to perform the many complex tasks it's entrusted with. Old science claims that those calories need to come from glucose (carbohydrates). Before going to the new science, let me ask you this:

What did the caveman do when he didn't find any food for days?

How did he hunt "the next meal" if he didn't have his minimum 130 g of carbohydrates to fuel his brain?

How could he be mentally sharp and have the physical strength to hunt his next meal?

I'm not trying to be sarcastic, I'm using critical thinking and logic to question what we are told.

I don't just accept it. I invite you to check if it makes sense from all perspectives. Use ancestral knowledge and modern nutrition to draw meaningful conclusions that will help you make the best choices to support your health and healing.

Now, let's see what modern science tells us.

The brain is our most energy demanding organ and is like a sensor that detects the most subtle drop in available fuels. The fuels available to us humans are glucose, ketones and free fatty acids. The brain can use as fuel either glucose or ketone bodies.[22] See Diagram #14. What the brain can't use are free fatty acids; they can't pass through the blood brain barrier to get into the brain. In fact, the brain can meet most of its energy needs from ketone bodies, in the context of restricted dietary carbohydrates or prolonged fasting. Skeletal muscles on the other hand can use all three substrates.

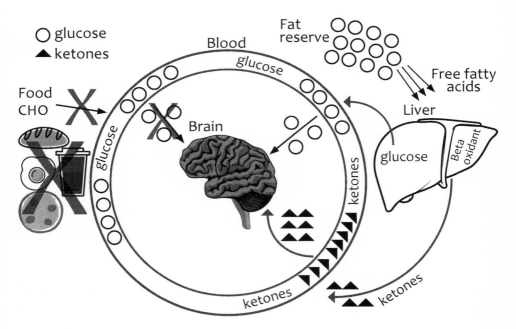

Diagram #14: Brain's energy sources.

Think of it this way: if glucose is available, the body, including the brain, will use it. When glucose is in short supply, the body taps into reserves and gets its energy from there. The reserves of energy are the small glycogen tank and the large fat tank. Regarding the brain, for as long as there is fuel available whether is glucose or ketone bodies, "the brain is happy," and it will not send any emergency messages out. You will have energy, and won't crash or hit the wall.

I hope this helps you understand that there is no minimum required amount of carbohydrates we need in order to survive, or for the brain to function at its highest capacity. We are designed to use more than one fuel and to switch from one to another based on availability. You will come across papers, blogs, and books that talk about metabolic flexibility. That's what *"metabolic flexibility"* is, the ability to shift energy metabolism from burning (oxidizing) carbohydrate to burning fat. Another term that is also often used is *"fat adapted."* What that means is the person's metabolism has adapted to oxidizing fat as fuel.

How long does it take for the body to adapt to less carbs and to switch energy metabolism from oxidizing glucose to oxidizing fat?

It doesn't happen overnight. It takes, on average, 3-4 weeks, and it happens faster if carbohydrate restriction is accompanied by fasting (prolonged or intermittent).

How many carbohydrates should you consume to achieve fat adaptation?

It depends on your age, activity level, gender, metabolic health, physiological state and degree of insulin resistance. This is where you need to personalize it to your unique needs.

According to Dr. Volek and Dr. Phinney, most individuals that are carb intolerant (aka. have insulin resistance) respond positively when they restrict their carb intake to less than 50 grams a day. That forces the body to enter the "fat burning mode," where it begins to mobilize fat from adipose tissue to supply the body with energy.

This is how I see it: when you eat less than 50 g of carbs in a day, it is like taking a metabolic trip in time, all the way to the caveman days. To survive, you have to turn off the "modern, 21st century metabolism" that runs on sugar and to switch back on the "ancestral metabolism" that runs on fat.

Do not panic! If you don't know how many carbs you eat currently, or you know and 50 g seems an impossible number to aim for, later in the book, under the Metabolic Reset Protocol, I include the steps to help you jumpstart your low carb, whole food journey.

The most important take home message is that the more weight you'll need to lose, the more severe your metabolic imbalance is. The more severe the insulin resistance is, the more carb intolerant you are. The more you restrict those carbs, the faster you'll see results.

So far we have reviewed foods sources of carbohydrates, what makes some foods more insulinogenic than others, what fiber is, and the concept of net carbs.

I didn't mention anything about portion size or grams of carbohydrates per serving of food, such as:

- one serving of rice is ⅓ of a cup and contains 15 g of carbs.

I did that on purpose, not because it's not important. It is. In fact, for many individuals it boils down to counting NC and maintaining it at a certain level in order to see lasting results. However, I feel that there is no need for you to memorize serving sizes and grams of carbs—you can always *"ask google"* when you don't know it. At one point on your low carb journey, it may be necessary for you to weigh your food and to log it in a nutrition app. That will help you easily figure out the grams of total carbs and net carbs as well as the rest of the macros in your food. With time, you will know it even without having to weigh it or log it. Practice makes perfect.

My main intention is to help you understand the basics, the fundamental principles of the low carb-high fat eating. Once you know without having to overthink what foods make it on your plate, whether you are eating at home or out at a restaurant; once you are ready to embrace it as your new life and eating style, then you will move to the fine tuning stage. You will look at portions, grams, and macronutrient ratios. And even that is temporary. After a while, you know it intuitively and instinctively, just like breathing or brushing your teeth.

If you are a type 2 or type 1 diabetic, then you will need to always monitor closely the macronutrient ratios, and the carbohydrate content of your meals alongside your blood sugar and ketones.

This concludes the knowledge-base on the first macronutrient, carbohydrates 101. Next let's talk about protein.

PROTEIN

3.2 PROTEIN 101.
HOW MUCH IS TOO MUCH AND WHY?

- Food sources

- Energetic value

- Main role in the body

- How much is too much and why!

- Protein, premature aging and chronic disease. Understanding the mTHOR pathway

Food sources and energetic value.

Protein is the second macronutrient found in food. We find protein in all food sources, both animal and plant.

Protein is made of many amino acids bound together. I like to think of proteins as necklaces made of pearls, which fold and take many shapes and forms. Each pearl represents an amino acid.

Unlike carbohydrates, proteins are nutritionally essential. That is due to the fact that there are 9 amino acids that the body must acquire from food sources in order to synthesize its own proteins.

- Protein in animal foods is always accompanied by fat and cholesterol;

- Animal foods don't contain dietary fiber;

- Muscle meat contains glycogen, the equivalent of plant starch; however, it is not absorbed in our body as a carbohydrate;

- Animal proteins are *"complete"* proteins, meaning they supply all 9 essential amino acids;

- Plant protein is less bioavailable than animal protein, which means it's more difficult to absorb it. The amino acids from plants are trapped inside the plant cells by fiber and others plant compounds that make digestion and absorption harder;

- Protein in plants is always accompanied by carbohydrates: starches, simple sugars and fiber. Because of this, plant proteins need to be looked at as insulinogenic foods; and

- Very few plant proteins are complete proteins, e.g. chia and hemp seeds, quinoa and soy. Following a strictly plant-based diet requires proper meal planning to make sure all the essential amino acids are supplied.

Good animal sources of protein are:

- eggs, meat, poultry, fish, seafood and cheese.

All plants contain protein. Some are a better source than others. For example,

- legumes are a better source of protein than fruits. They have higher protein content than carbohydrates; and

- Nuts and seeds are the best source of plant protein for someone that wants to follow the therapeutic low carbohydrate diet we've been talking about. Most nuts are low in carbohydrates and high in fats, with moderate protein content. They are a great flour substitute in cooking and baking to replace grain flours. For the complete list of nuts please see the Resources section of this book.

When following a low carb eating plan, it's best and easier to meet your protein needs from animal foods. Consuming plant protein, such as beans or other legumes, grains or starches, will trigger an insulin response that will hinder your goal of keeping insulin low and reversing IR. That's not to say that if you choose to eat a plant-based diet you can't follow the low carb, high fat nutritional ketosis plan. With proper planning, you can.

Energetic Value of Protein.

- Just like carbohydrates, protein also provides 4 calories per gram.

Main Roles of Protein for the Human Body.

From all three macronutrients found in food, protein is the only one that is not used as fuel for the body. As long as we continue to eat and the body has access to carbohydrates, protein and fats, it will preferentially use carbohydrates and fat as fuel over protein.

So, what's the role of protein in the body?

The importance of protein in health and nourishment can't be overlooked. The word protein originates from the Greek word "proteos," which means primary or taking first place. Proteins serve a structural role. From muscles to hair, we are made out of protein. Enzymes are made of protein molecules and are required by most human physiological processes from digestion, to blood coagulation and muscle contraction. The immune system produces immunoglobulin (aka. antibodies), which are also made out of protein. There are transport proteins, which, just as their name implies, act as carriers and move substances, minerals, vitamins and oxygen throughout the body (e.g. albumin, hemoglobin).

An interesting fact about proteins is that, due to their amino acid composition, they can act as a buffer in the body. They buffer or modulate the changes in pH in the body. As you've probably heard, people talk about keeping your body alkaline. Take it with a grain of salt. Our body has different pH in different tissues.

Blood pH for example ranges from 7.35 to 7.45, while cellular pH is more acidic (e.g. the pH of muscle cells is 6.9). Amino acids can act as an acid or as a base by accepting or donating hydrogen ions and helping to keep the pH normal.

We also see proteins binding to molecules of sugars to form glycoproteins, found usually in body secretions like mucus and connective tissues like collagen and elastin. We find glycoproteins as part of the hormone structure as well.

Proteins also have the ability to bind to fat and create lipoproteins which are like transport molecules for fat and cholesterol.

As you can see, proteins play many vital roles in the body, from structure to function. They truly are essential for our survival.

It is well known that protein plays a big role in weight loss, but how does it do that?

Protein:

1. has a higher thermogenic effect , meaning the body expends more energy to digest protein versus fat or carbohydrates. This is known as the thermogenic effect of food (TEF);

2. stays longer in the stomach, which increases the feeling of satiety. You feel full for a longer time; hence, you don't need to eat as often; and

3. when part of a mixed meal that contains fat (e.g. butter, olive oil) and non-insulinogenic carbs (e.g broccoli, avocado, leafy greens), it stimulates the release of glucagon, and favors a metabolic environment that promotes fat burning rather than fat storage. So, it makes a huge difference what you have your steak with: broccoli and kale with plenty of olive oil, versus mash potatoes, bread or fries.

Now, the question is how much protein should you eat? Is it possible to eat too much protein?

HDL and LDL Lipoproteins

Protein binds to lipids, forming lipoproteins. This is a very important function proteins play in the body. Let's see why.

Protein can be by itself in the blood, but fat can't, so protein comes to its rescue.

Have you ever tried to mix water with oil? Were you successful? No! Why not? Because water and fat don't mix together. Fat is hydrophobic; it can't mix with water.

The way we can mix water with fat is to add a third party agent that acts as a mediator, on one side (the water side) it is water friendly and on the other side (the fat side) it is fat friendly. Protein is like that: it's both water and fat friendly.

Let me give you an example of a lipoprotein. LDL and HDL cholesterol are lipoproteins.

The only way we can transport cholesterol, and fats (which are water phobic) through blood (which is a water-like medium) is to pack them in a carrier that loves water (is hydrophilic). And that is the lipoproteins system.

Imagine those lipoproteins like balls, which in their core keep fats and cholesterol, and the outside is made of proteins. [19]

That's how cholesterol is transported throughout the body, in lipoproteins called Low Density Lipoproteins (LDL) and High Density Lipoproteins (HDL). The difference between the two is their density and their destination. LDL is going from the liver to the cells, while HDL is transported from the cells to the liver. Saying that one is good and the other one is bad is like saying that the plane that takes you from New York to LA is the bad and the one that brings you from LA to New York is the good one.

Labeling lipoproteins as atherogenic is a complex process and has to take into account multiple factors, such as particle size, oxidation, inflammatory markers, and fibrinogen, just to name a few.

How Much Protein is too Much and Why?

There is a very common misconception that a low carbohydrate diet is an *"all you can eat meat diet."* That couldn't be further from the truth. I don't want to point fingers, but the Paleo diet is one of them (a little too high in protein and not low enough in carbs). Nevertheless, a Paleo-like diet approach helps at first, as it removes all processed foods, grains and some starches; however, long term it's another story.

First, let's see how you can determine your unique protein needs and then I'll explain what the possible pitfalls of eating too much protein long term are. Occasionally it's fine to have more protein and more food overall; it is like going from feast to famine.

Current dietary allowance (RDA) for protein intake is 0.8 g per kg of body weight per day for adults. Athletes, children, adolescents, pregnant and lactating women require more.

At first when the body is adapting to using fat as fuel, the requirement for protein is slightly higher, and intuitively most people will consume a higher amount of protein. Once the body is well adapted to using fat as the primary source of fuel, in the context of a low carbohydrate intake, the need for protein diminishes, while the fat content of the diet rises to meet the person's energy demands.

Dr. Voleck, in his book "The Art and Science of Low Carbohydrate Performance," recommends a range of 0.6 – 1 gram per pound of lean body mass (1.3 - 2.2 g per kg of lean body mass). This seems like a broad range, but it takes into account activity level. The higher range applies to individuals that are more active, as they have higher needs for protein.[42]

I am a little more conservative in my protein estimates, for me personally as well as for most of my clients. I'm using 1-1.5 g of protein per Kg lean body mass per day.

There are several ways in which you can calculate your lean muscle mass and percent of body fat. Later, in the Fats 101 section, I talk more about body composition.

Since protein has more of a functional and structural role than of a fuel role, it makes sense to eat only as much protein as is needed for the body to maintain its function and structure. Excess amino acids can and will be used to produce glucose. That's why it's best to base calculations on lean body weight and not total body weight.

I will use my own body as an example to illustrate:

I weigh 57 kg (57X2.2 = 125 lbs.). That is total body weight.

I have an estimated FFMM (fat free muscle mass - includes muscles, bones and blood) of 45 kg (90 lbs.).

Using the above formula 45X1 = 45 g of protein per day, or 6-7 oz.

That includes protein from eggs, cheese, meats, fish, nuts, seeds, and other low carb plant foods. As you can see, it is a small amount, smaller than most trainers would tell me I need. If I am using Dr. Volek's recommendation, my protein intake would range from 54 to 90 g of protein/day. During my heavier training days, when I get ready for a long bike event (75-100 miles), I consume more protein, close to the upper range (70-90 g/day). It happens naturally, instinctively. But, outside of that, I average about 50 g of protein a day. I have been maintaining my weight and my muscle mass as mentioned above for the past couple of years, probably longer, but that's when I started keeping track of it.

Now, of course, I'm *"a study of one."* I'm not saying what's working for me will work for you nor am I telling you to do exactly what I'm doing. You will need to determine what works for you.

On a side note: I measure my body composition using a Tanita scale. This scale uses body impedance technology and provides total body weight as well as percent body fat, percent water and calculated fat free muscle mass (FFMM) in kilograms or pounds. It is, of course, an estimate, as it is not the most accurate method to use to assess body composition. However, doing it always at the same time of the day, under the same circumstances, on the same scale, provides a good level of reliability. It helps me see my weight and body composition trends over time.

> *Is eating more protein helping you gain more muscle?*
>
> *To build muscle mass, you need to stimulate the muscles with exercise. It is the tear and repair of the muscle that happens during exercise, followed by an adequate intake of quality protein, that supports muscle growth.*

Why more is not better when it comes to food in general and protein in particular?

To understand this next part, I would like to use an example. Let's pretend you just bought a new blender. The blender's life expectancy, as per the manufacturer, is 20 years. After 20 years it is expected that it will break and you will need to get a new one. The manufacturer tells you during these 20 years, you will need to change some parts and to do periodic maintenance or resets. The blades, the containers, something in the engine, etc. will need upkeep. The manufacturer is nice and gives you a seven-year warranty for your 20-year product. You, the owner of the blender, are now in charge of how you use the blender, and how and when you will change defective parts while the blender is still under warranty. This will allow you to fully use the blender up to the 20 years, as indicated by the manufacturer.

How does this relate to our body and the food we eat?

We're going to pretend that each cell in our body is the blender from our analogy. The average human is made of 30 trillion cells. [23] Each cell comes with a predetermined lifespan. In other words, each cell has a predetermined, genetically encoded death. There is a continuous turnover of our body's cells and tissues. The pre-programmed cellular death is called apoptosis. That is the equivalent of the 20-year lifespan of the blender. Just as you have to change some parts of your blender to make sure it functions well for the 20 years, so do our cells; they need regular maintenance. Periodically, we have to get rid of cellular components that become damaged within the cells. This assures that the cells function well and reach their genetically encoded lifespan.

This maintenance process is called autophagy. Auto=self, Phagia =eating. *"The body eats itself away."* Well, kind of; it gets rid of cellular junk, which, if not cleared away, can potentially impair the function of the cell, the tissues, organs, and, eventually, the whole body.

Let's summarize it:

- Apoptosis = cellular death (genetically preprogramed)

- Autophagy = cellular cleaning (periodic, volunteer maintenance)

Now you may be asking what turns on or off autophagy, and what protein has to do with any of these?

There is a metabolic pathway called mTOR. It stands for mechanistic target of rapamycin (or mammalian target of rapamycin). This metabolic pathway was relatively newly discovered (late 90s) during research done on rapamycin as a potent anti-cancer therapy. It turns out that mTOR controls autophagy. When it is turned on, it blocks or it stops autophagy. When it's suppressed, autophagy is turned on.

What controls mTOR? Nutrients from food and hormones. To be more exact amino acids, insulin, and growth factors, which are all produced when we eat. [24]

Fasting is the best way to suppress mTOR and to initiate autophagy, but there is another way of doing it. That is a well-designed low carbohydrate, low to moderate protein and high fat diet. Once again, fat stays neutral; it doesn't seem to interfere with mTOR, just as it doesn't interfere with the metabolic hormones. Don't you think that it's time that we *make peace with fat*?

I like to think of the mTOR as a switch or a sensor.

When we eat, primarily carbs and protein, mTOR is stimulated and it turns off the *"self-eating"* program, the autophagy. Stimulated mTOR means the body is ready to build new tissues, to grow and reproduce, as in time of abundance. Diagram #15 below illustrates it well:

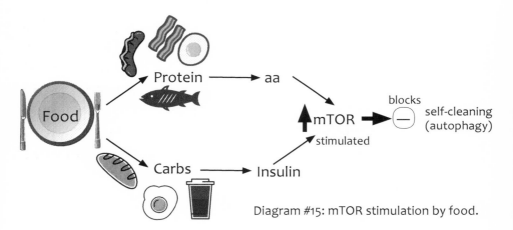

Diagram #15: mTOR stimulation by food.

In the absence of nutrients (glucose, amino acids), and when insulin is kept low, the *"self-cleaning"* program is turned on and the body enters a "cellular and mitochondrial detox," as in times of scarcity. This detox is slightly different from the humoral-liver detox most people think of when they hear the word "detox," like in a juice cleanse, for example.

- mTOR is suppressed during fasting and that's when the deep cellular detox happens at its best.

Diagram #16: mTOR inhibition during fasting.

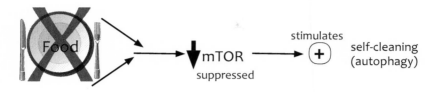

mTOR is a wonderful built-in mechanism that is of incredible benefit to young growing bodies and athletes. They are in greater need for growth, recovery and strength. Stimulating the mTOR pathway with food assures that. For young growing children and athletes, it makes sense to eat more protein, carbs, and even to eat more often.

For the aging body, and the ill body, which have accumulated lots of cellular and mitochondrial damage, the mTOR serves more when it is suppressed. Imagine that the aging body or the ill body has filled up the trash can with *"cellular junk."* What do you do when the trash is full in your house? You take the trash out before it begins to stink up the whole house. What do you do to take out cellular junk, to initiate self-cleaning? You want to suppress mTOR. You engage in periodic fasting and follow a low carbohydrate moderate protein diet.

If you want to be proactive, to prevent premature aging, inflammation and degenerative diseases, you can act before "the trashcan gets full."

> *Against common nutrition advice!*
>
> *Eating every 2-3 hours is not speeding up your metabolism and helping you lose weight. It is "keeping the trash in" and adding more to it. Also, eating a high carbohydrate, high protein diet is not helping your body to repair itself.*
>
> *Unless you are a growing kid (that's not overweight or obese), eating all the time, "grazing," or having 6 small meals a day, is not the best strategy for weight loss, diabetes management, reversal of metabolic disorders, or premature aging.*
>
> *Eating less often, fasting and eating a low carb, high fat, and adequate protein diet may prevent premature aging, cancer, and reverse metabolic disorders by allowing your body to self-clean on a regular basis.*

Another reason to keep protein intake just right is its gluconeogenic effect. When you consume more protein than what your body needs for its own maintenance, repair, growth, and function, the excess amino acids are directed to the liver and converted into glucose, in the process of gluconeogenesis. If the glucose levels rise too high, insulin is released to bring glucose down, and, if you recall, when insulin is elevated, fat burning stops. Therefore, you are unable to enter or stay in the magical zone of nutritional ketosis, and you can't fully benefit from the effects of ketone bodies.

This aspect is particularly important for people that use keto diets as means to starve cancer, as well as for those with neurodegenerative diseases. More about ketones will come in the Fat 101 section.

One last reason why eating just the right amount of protein matters is the fact that protein digestion leads to nitrogen production through a metabolic pathway that involves the kidney and the liver, and ammonia is produced and is eliminated from the body via urine. If too much protein is consumed, especially if you have a predisposition to kidney disease, it can affect kidney function.

A Word about Protein Quality.

Just as it is important to get your vegetables from trusted sources (preferably organic locally grown and not genetically modified), when it comes to the animal protein, quality is just as important as quantity. When I say quality protein, I mean foods from animals that are raised by small farmers in humane conditions, free-range on green pastures under the sunlight, eating grass as their natural food and not fed genetically modified corn and soybean crops. They are not treated with heavy doses of antibiotics, growth hormones, steroids or any other drugs.

Why is this important?

Just as we are what we eat, absorb, and store, so are the animals that become our food. I'm talking here not only about the humanitarian aspect of raising and slaughtering animals, which I definitely care about—that's why I don't eat animal food if I don't know the small farm it is coming from. Hint: when I eat out, I become a vegetarian again, as most animal foods (including fish) at restaurants comes from confinement farming, also known as CAFOs (confinement animal feeding operations).

The nutritional composition of pasture-raised animal products is far superior to those that are raised in confinement. For example, meat from grass-fed animals and eggs from free range chickens have higher doses of vitamin D and omega-3 fatty acids.

Another aspect to keep in mind is that animals, just like us, store toxins in the adipose tissue. When eating animal products (fat, meats, organs) from animals that were given growth hormones, antibiotics, steroid drugs, etc. to survive their unsanitary living conditions, and to speed up their growth and development, it has an impact on the quality of that animal food and, as an extension, on our health.

Fish and seafood are also to be purchased carefully. Avoid farm raised fish as it is the equivalent of the confinement raised animals. They are raised in crowded ponds, fed food pellets that are not their natural food in their natural environment, treated with antibiotics and other drugs. Even wild caught fish can be a problem, as the oceans are polluted and so are the fish that live in the ocean. It's sad and scary to even think about this, but when you eat fish you are at risk of polluting your body with mercury and persistent organic pollutants (POP).

A study published in the Journal of Science Advances found that environmental pollutants present in fish interfere with the human body's natural defense system to expel harmful toxins.[32] Keep in mind, the larger the fish, the more contaminated it is, as it feeds on all the other fishes, and it lives longer hence it accumulates more pollutants in its body (e.g. shark fish, tuna fish, sea bass, etc.).

There are many online resources you can use to help you select fish and seafood that is the least contaminated and environmentally friendly fished.

Small fish like sardines, herring, mackerel and anchovy are your best choices from all perspectives. I always have a stock of sardines in my house. I buy them in water, then, if I need to, I add my own olive oil to it. I drink the brine they are coming with (I love the salt in it). My favorite brand is Wild Planet and they pack their sardines in BPA (bisphenol-a) free cans, which is also important when it comes to toxins from the environment.

You may say, "Mihaela, the meat, eggs and cheese that comes from the local farmers, or the wild caught fish, is 5 times more expensive as the meat I can buy at my local grocery store." I know it! I see that, too. Yet, I make a choice. I choose to invest my money in my health, in disease prevention and not in disease care. I also choose to support local small farms. The way I see it, there are only two options: either I pay more on food now, by investing in what matters to me the most—my health, my energy, my mental and physical body—or I pay later in doctor's visits, prescription drugs, hospitalization, assisted living, etc.

This concludes the section on protein. Next, let's talk about how to make peace with fat and why.

My "MUST".

I choose to buy food from local farmers.
I never question their prices, because I know the hard work that goes into growing vegetables and raising animals.
I believe I'm worth the investment.
I believe, I vote with my $$, hence I choose to support small local farmers.
I value the most: my health, my body and my energy.
That's my "MUST."
Tony Robbins says, "People always meet their musts." And he's right.

Do you know your musts?

When I pay more for the meats or the vegetables that come from a local farmer, I do it with a big smile. I imagine the ripple effect. I can see how this helps farmers get stronger. I see more of us making a stand and supporting small local farmers. I see them becoming, once again, the primary food provider for us, rather than the big corporations. As the small farmers grow stronger we get healthier, with each bite of food we take. Food becomes our medicine and our preventive measure.

I felt compelled to share with you my life's philosophy, my core belief and what I stand for. I can't bring a number based argument against the fact that, yes, you need to pay more for quality food. The only argument I can bring to the table is my belief. All I want is to share "me" with you; my healing journey, my knowledge, my passion and my core beliefs.

My deepest desire remains to raise your awareness, to empower you with knowledge and to help you build up your belief, so that you go and take action.

You show up every day. You set up one goal each day. You strengthen your belief each day. You act on it each day. You succeed each day. And that's how magic happens! One day at a time, day after day!

Proteins At a Glance.

☐   Proteins are essential and vital for human life.

☐   We get protein from all foods. However, the best source of bio-available amino acids and complete proteins are those of animal origin.

☐   Animal protein is accompanied by fat, and not by carbs so this favors a fat burning metabolism. One exception to this rule is milk.

☐   When it comes to protein, more is not better. It is important to match protein intake to your unique bodily needs based on your lean body weight, age, activity level and physiological state (growing, pregnant, postmenopausal).

☐   A guideline to use when calculating your protein needs is 0.6-1 g protein per pound of lean body weight per day.

☐   When you first start the low carbohydrate therapeutic eating, your protein requirements are higher while going through the adaptation phase for about 3-4 weeks, and up to few months. Afterwards, you will benefit more from keeping protein intake at low to moderate levels.

☐   Excess amino acids from protein digestion turn on the mTOR pathway and hinder autophagy, your body's *"self-eating"* ability.

☐   Excess amino acids from protein digestion can be converted into glucose and affect fat burning metabolism.

☐   Quality of protein is just as important, if not more, than the quantity.

FAT

3.3 FAT 101:
MAKE PEACE WITH FAT

- Not all fats are created equal:

    - Natural and manmade fats

    - Saturated fat and cholesterol, should you fear them?

- Fats 101-energy, properties and food sources

- Nutritional ketosis VS diabetic ketoacidosis.

- Ketone bodies, what are they and are they harming you?

Fat continues to be a hot and controversial topic. Especially when it comes to saturated fat and cholesterol; there seems to be a war going on. They were demonized for making us fat and causing diabetes and heart disease. They were removed from our plate and replaced with carbs, vegetable oils and margarines. There is no secret that this particular approach, which was promoted and followed by the majority of our population for the past 50 years, didn't help us lose weight, nor did it reduce the rates of diabetes and cardiovascular diseases.

If anything, the numbers have been consistently and progressively going up.

My intention is to help you understand what role fat in general—and saturated fats and cholesterol in particular—play in our body, from function to structure. Why eating fat doesn't make you fat. How you can make fat your primary source of energy and, of course, what are the fats to love and the fats to ditch?

My hope is that by the end of this chapter you will not only make peace with fat, but actually fall in love with it. It is the hardest dietary change you will probably have to make. I see it every day with my clients. It is so ingrained in their brain (as it may be in yours) that *"fat is bad"* that it takes months to drop that belief, to release from our fear of fats and to embrace the fact that fats are our biggest friend when it comes to losing weight, getting healthier, having lasting energy, breaking free of food cravings, and healing.

Are you ready to change your knowledge and mind set about fat, so you can change what you eat to improve your health and life?

Is it high fat or low carb we are talking about in this book?

In the context of a low carbohydrate, moderate protein diet, fat—the third macronutrient we get from food—comes in the greatest amount. So, we could be talking about this therapeutic way of eating as a high fat diet instead of a low carb diet. I'm afraid most people would freak out at the thought that they can eat, or that they can benefit from, a high fat diet. That's why I and most practitioners out there presented it as a low carbohydrate diet, rather than a high fat diet. Both are true. In fact, a high fat, high carb diet would be a real metabolic disaster, and that's pretty much what the standard American diet, also known as SAD, is.

Since we are going to talk about fat, and a high fat diet, let's make sure we address the quality of it too.

Yes, it matters what fat you eat, as they are not all created equal. When we talk about fats, we usually refer to their physical structure and properties. We look at them as saturated fats, unsaturated (mono and polyunsaturated) fats, trans-fats and cholesterol. That's all important and I will come back to it, but for now let's look at fat through a different eye.

The way I want to talk about fats next is slightly different and I believe somewhat simpler. It has to do with the way they are made.

Natural and Manmade Fats.

Natural fats are part of whole foods, both plant and animal.

Plant sources of natural fats are:

- avocado, olives, nuts, seeds, coconut, cacao nibs.

Animal sources of natural fats are:

- muscle meats and organ meats of 4 legged animals, as well as poultry, fish, seafood, and eggs.

Manmade fats are extracted as oils or butters from a whole food. They can be split in two categories:

- stone-made

- industry-made

Stone-made fats are extracts from a whole food in a relatively easy, effortless way. It doesn't require a factory, a specialized complicated refinery, or distillery to be made, as the industry-made fats do. They are usually extracted using methods such as cold pressing, centrifugation and low temperature melting.

Examples of these type of fats are:

- olive oil, coconut oil/butter, cacao butter, flaxseed and hemp oils;

- lard (pork fat), tallow (beef fat), and any fat that comes from cooking/roasting, chicken, goose, duck;

- fish fat (we mostly get this as a fish oil supplement and, although this is a refined product, it has its role and place in our healing), and whale fat; and

- butter, ghee, sweet heavy cream and sour cream.

All of the above fats are good, healing, energy giving fats. You may incorporate them in your diet without fear or guilt.

The industry-made fats are another story. Let's see what those are and why they are not on your shopping list, in your cupboard or on your plate (unless you eat out a lot, as it's hard to find restaurants that use natural fats).

You know when you walk down the aisle of the supermarket that has oils and vinegar? That's where you find the industry-made oils.

- vegetable oils, such as corn, soybean, peanut, canola oils; and

- margarines and other vegetable spreads.

I'm sure you are asking, "Why not these oils, Mihaela?"

Vegetable oils are highly refined "food-like substances." In order to extract oil from corn or soybean, as an example, you need to subject them to high temperatures and chemical solvents to remove their color and odor. The end product—an odorless, flavorless, tasteless oil—is far from being healthy.

There are numerous scientific studies that show a correlation between the consumption of these oils and the incidence of cancer, heart disease, diabetes and other inflammatory related conditions.

These oils are polyunsaturated fats, which means they are extremely sensitive to the action of heat, light and oxygen. When cooking with them, they get oxidized and become damaged. Consuming them contributes to oxidative damage and inflammatory processes in the body. They are a high source of omega-6 fats (the inflammatory fats). A good ratio of the omega-6 to omega-3 fats is 2:1 or 3:1. Our modern diet today supplies us with a ratio of 15:1 or as high as 20:1. How is that possible? This is the direct result of increased consumption of vegetable oils and all the processed foods made with them.

Take a look at the ingredients in any packaged food you buy (potato chips, tortilla chips, pita chips, crackers, cookies, breads, cakes, etc.). You'll always find one of these ingredients: canola oil, corn, soybean or sunflower oil, etc. Things get even more complicated if those fats are hydrogenated or partially hydrogenated.

What about margarines and vegetable spreads?

It is obvious they are man-made products as well. Margarines are made by adding hydrogen molecules to the unsaturated carbon atoms of fatty acids found in vegetable oils. By doing this, they turn from liquid to solid and behave like saturated fats. They are solid at room temperature, more heat stable and can be used in cooking instead of lard, tallow or butter. This process is called hydrogenation or partial hydrogenation. It leads to the solidification of oils.

Margarines are solid vegetable oils. If the vegetable oils in their liquid form are not good for us, will their solid form be good?

They behave like saturated fats, but they are not and they don't have cholesterol, so they must be good. Well, here's the catch: in the process of hydrogenation their isomeric structure (special orientation) changes from "cis" to "trans," and they become trans-fatty acids. Cis form is the natural orientation of fats, the way they are found in foods, while trans is not. In nature we find only a small amount of trans-fatty acids in the animal products or ruminates, as they are the result of microbial fermentation in the rumen.[52] The main sources of trans-fatty acids are margarines, shortening, frying fats, and all processed foods (from baked goods to cookies).

What About Canola Oil? Isn't That Healthy?

This is my favorite question of all.

Canola oil is a rich source of the omega-3 anti-inflammatory fats. So, you might assume canola oil is good for you. Let's see.

By virtue of being a polyunsaturated fat, canola oil is not suitable for cooking, as it easily gets damaged by heat, oxygen and light. But that's not the only reason to avoid canola oil.

We know that olive oil is extracted from olives and coconut oil from coconut, but what about canola oil? There is no canola seed or fruit out there. Canola oil is extracted from the seed of the plant rapeseed that's been modified by Canadian scientists to make it non-toxic. Yes, there is no food out there called canola. The name Canola is a manmade name (just as the oil is). It's a combination of the words Canada and oil.

The original rapeseed plant and its oil are toxic to humans. It had long been used for industrial purposes before the Canadians decided to "play" with it and to make it edible. Talk about a massively produced Franken-food!

The rapeseed plant has a high erucic acid content. Erucic acid is toxic to humans and animals; in rats it causes fatty degeneration of the heart, kidney, adrenals and thyroid. [35, 36] The Canadian scientists, through hybridization methods, created a rapeseed plant with low erucic acid content, which allows the extraction of what we know today as canola oil. Although canola oil may be low enough in erucic acid to prevent its toxic effects, it doesn't make it a natural fat, nor a good choice when it comes to health.

The bottom line is: canola oil is extracted from a plant that doesn't even exist naturally. It's a man-made product from start to finish; a "food-like substance."

Take It To The Supermarket!

When you read food labels and you see hydrogenated ... oil or partially hydrogenated ... oil you probably know that's not a good choice.

By adding hydrogen to oils, through the process of hydrogenation, trans-fatty acids are created. It is well accepted that trans-fats are detrimental to cardiovascular and metabolic health. The FDA requires food manufacturers to list the amount of trans-fats found in the food on the nutritional facts label.

HINT: The nutrients listed on the food label are based on one serving, not on the entire package. More often than not, there is more than one serving per package. You must see what the serving size is and how many servings are in the package.

If the amount of trans-fats is less than 0.5 g/serving, they will be listed as 0 g.

For example, if you were to consume 2 of 10 or more servings of a food that has 0.4 g/serving, the amount rises to well above the minimum acceptable dose of 0.5 g, to levels high enough to cause harm. Yet, it will be listed as 0 g of trans-fats.

Aside from looking at the nutrition label, it is important that you read the ingredients list. It is best to avoid buying any food that lists hydrogenated or partially hydrogenated oils as one of its ingredients. Usually you see these on chips, cookies, crackers, bread etc. Just about any processed package food is made using some form of vegetable oil or hydrogenated fats.

Final Thoughts About Fat Quality.

You know I like to stop and look back at how our ancestors ate, especially when it comes to foods that are controversial today, as it raises many questions in my mind.

Our ancestors were eating pretty much the entire animal—that included its fat and cholesterol. They ate natural fats. Sometime later in human history, tropical fats, like coconut oil, and Mediterranean fats, such as olive oil, were added to the diet. The era of man-made fats began.

However, people didn't have access to margarines or vegetable oils until very recent in human history. With the industrialized era, the food available to us changed drastically, and industry-made oils were added. The era of processed foods began and the human health started to decline.

My hope is that I am able to bring home the message and to advocate for the fats that come as part of whole foods, and that, if you choose an oil or butter extracted by man, the extraction method is not of the industrialized era.

In conclusion: eat natural fat and stay away from industry-made fats like vegetable oils and margarines

Fat, Saturated Fat and Cholesterol: Should You Fear Them?

The fat craze began around the 1950s when the diet-heart hypothesis was formulated by Ancel Keys. He managed to show that there was a correlation between the type and the amount of fats and cholesterol consumed, and the incidence of heart disease.

Dr. Natasha Campbell-McBride in her book, "Put Your Heart in Your Mouth," states: *"It is completely baffling as to why on earth the scientific community at that time accepted this kind of scientific evidence."* [25]

Sadly, even today, mainstream medicine doesn't fully accept the inaccuracy of the diet-heart hypothesis. This probably explains why there is so much conflicting information about fats. You may hear from your doctor that saturated fats and cholesterol are bad for you, therefore you should avoid them. While other practitioners, such as Dr. Perlmutter, the author of "the Grain Brain" and the Brain Maker books, invites us to bring the butter back. Books such are "Eat Fat Get Thin," authored by Dr. Mark Hyman, and "Fat For Fuel," by Dr. Joseph Mercola are also shining light on the controversial issues of fats, saturated fats and cholesterol.

To help you make peace with fat, let's look at the many roles fat and cholesterol play in human health and body function.

Fats are essential nutrients.

There are two classes of fatty acids that are "essential," meaning we need to acquire them from our diet, as our body can't manufacture them.

- Omega-3 (alpha linoleic acid ALA) and

- Omega-6 (gamma linolenic acid GLA).

I introduced them when we talked about low grade, silent inflammation. They are the main ingredient the body uses to produce pro and anti-inflammatory eicosanoids.

Fats play a structural and functional role in the human body. They are important components of all cell membranes. Together with cholesterol, they help the cells form and maintain their structure, and confer just the right flexibility.

Every cell membrane contains saturated and polyunsaturated fats and cholesterol. The proportions in which we find them in the cell membrane is crucial to cell function and structure. Some cells and organs are richer in fats than others. The brain, for example, is 60% fat by weight and our nerves are covered with a substance called myelin that's made of 40% cholesterol.

Think of cholesterol as a stabilizing agent; it gets in between phospholipids and prevents the fats from clinging together. It makes the cell more firm. Too much cholesterol would make it too rigid and not enough would make it too fluid. Without cholesterol, the cell can't maintain shape and structure, and it would be runny, kind of like an egg white.

Note: Phospholipids are the way fats are found in the cell membrane: a lipid molecule bound to a phosphate group. See the image below, for a visual representation of the cell membrane and its phospholipid bilayer. The phosphate group is water-friendly, while the fat is water-phobic.

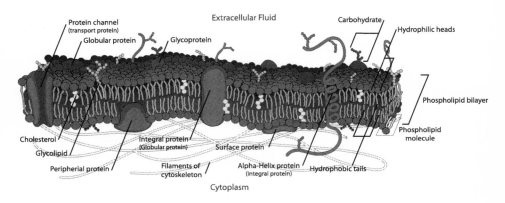

Steroid hormone production.

Fats and cholesterol are the substrates the body uses to produce steroid hormones (adrenal and gonadal hormones).

Vitamin D synthesis.

The cholesterol found in our skin, when it is exposed to the UVB sun rays, converts into vitamin D.

Absorption of fat soluble vitamins.

Fats are crucial for the absorption of fat soluble vitamins from our diet. Without fat, we can't absorb any other fatty substance (e.g. Coenzyme Q10 or vitamin A, D, E, or K).

Endocrine organ.

Fat behaves as an endocrine organ and produces hormones which regulate satiety. The one that gets the most attention is leptin. Obese individuals have high levels of leptin, yet their body is resistant to its action of suppressing the appetite. Leptin resistance and insulin resistance happen in the body usually at the same time. Weight loss, fat loss and low carb diets seem to help reverse leptin resistance as well.

Doesn't knowing the many roles fats play in the human body make you begin to look at fat with different, perhaps even a bit more loving, eyes?

Energetic Value of Fat.

- Fat provides 9 calories per g.

Types of Fats, Their Properties and Food Sources.

The way I like to classify fats is using four criteria as presented below:

- Saturated or unsaturated fats – refers to the amount of hydrogen molecules that occupy the carbon atoms of a fat

- Long, medium or short fats – refers to the number of carbon atoms that make the fatty acid chain (the length of the chains)

- Mono, di or tri glycerides – refers to the number of fatty acids that are bound to the glycerol bone

- Cis and trans-fatty acids – refers to their isomeric special orientation

White fat and brown fat!

Not all fat stored in your body is created equal! There are two types of fat: white and brown.

☐ White fat requires very little energy to be maintained. It's metabolically inert.

☐ Brown fat is metabolically very active. It requires, just like muscle, energy to be maintained. It has a very good blood supply and loads of mitochondria.

To understand what I mean by metabolically inert or metabolically active, let's talk about muscle tissue.

Muscle requires more energy from the body to maintain its function. Your basal metabolic rate (BMR) is greatly influenced by the muscle weight and not as much by fat. The higher your muscle mass is in relation to your total body weight, the better it is when it comes to health and weight management. Muscle is a very active and energy demanding tissue. The more muscle mass you have, the higher your BMR is going to be. This means you burn more calories at rest just to maintain those muscles. So, the ideal body composition is to have more muscle mass and less fat tissue.

From a health point of view this is very important, as a high body fat percentage, or obesity is a major risk factor for all metabolic and cardiovascular diseases.

See the body composition table for guidelines based on gender and activity levels.[37]

Body Fat Guidelines as Per American Council On Exercise

Classification	Female % Fat	Male % Fat
Acceptable	25-31	18-24
Fitness	21-24	14-17
Athletes	14-20	6-13
Essential	10-13	2-5
Obesity	32	25

Although it is desirable to have a low body fat percentage, what is even more important is to have more brown fat. Brown fat requires, just like muscle, energy to be maintained.

Not only that, but brown fat seems to waste some energy when it generates heat via thermogenesis (thermogenesis = dissipation of energy derived from ingested food). One of the main functions of brown fat is thermoregulation, or heat generation.[9]

Because it's a metabolically active tissue and it wastes energy, having more brown fat turns out to be a good thing when it comes to losing or maintaining weight.

Brown fat is called brown because it really looks brown. Its color is given by the high number of mitochondria. We are all born with brown fat. In fact, infants and children have the highest percent of brown fat. As we grow older, we lose most of the brown fat and accumulate more of the white fat. If you look at infants exposed to cold, they don't shiver. Do you know why? Because their brown fat generates heat and keeps them warm. As we age, we lose most of the brown fat and thermoregulation is taken over by the muscles. Adults exposed to cold begin to shiver and generate heat through muscle contractions. An interesting fact is that obese individuals seem to have less brown fat than leaner individuals.

Due to brown fat's ability to burn energy, researchers hope to find a way to use it to help people lose weight.

How do you gain more brown fat? It is known that cold exposure stimulates brown fat activity. It is quite popular to hear people practicing ice baths or cryotherapy (cryo-cold). You may say that that sounds good, but there is no way I'm going to submerge myself in ice baths. I say you don't have to, because the food you eat can help you make more of your white fat behave like brown fat.

When we eat in a way that keeps insulin levels low and fat is burned to produce ketones, it creates a metabolic environment which allows white fat to behave more like brown fat: it increase the numbers of mitochondria in white fat and it makes it a more metabolically active tissue. This has been seen in animal studies, and it has relevance to weight loss.

Benjamin Bickman, PhD, focuses his research on understanding insulin resistance, white and brown fat metabolism, and their contribution to chronic diseases. You can find more information about this emerging area of research on his website www. insuliniq.com.

In conclusion, aim to bring your body fat percentage in a healthy range. That in and of itself may help you make some of the white fat turn brown.

Just as proteins are found in all foods of plant and animal origin, so are fats. Fats come in many shapes, forms, flavors and colors.

It is worth mentioning here that cholesterol is not a fat, it is a wax, an ester of a fatty acid, and it can only be found in foods of animal origin.

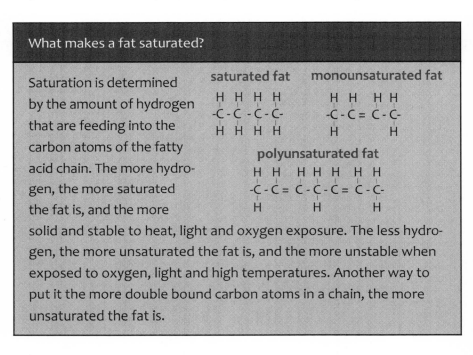

What makes a fat saturated?

Saturation is determined by the amount of hydrogen that are feeding into the carbon atoms of the fatty acid chain. The more hydrogen, the more saturated the fat is, and the more solid and stable to heat, light and oxygen exposure. The less hydrogen, the more unsaturated the fat is, and the more unstable when exposed to oxygen, light and high temperatures. Another way to put it the more double bound carbon atoms in a chain, the more unsaturated the fat is.

Saturated Fats (SF).

These are your best fats when it comes to high temperature cooking. Let's go through some of their physical properties so you know how to recognize them. This review will also help you understand why these are the best fats to use when it comes to high temperature cooking. **How Do You Recognize SF?**

- Solid at room temperature & solid in the refrigerator.

- More stable at high temperatures than unsaturated fats.

- Have a high smoking point, meaning the temperature at which they catch fire is high.

- Don't get easily denatured by high heat, oxygen and light.

- They have a longer shelf life and are more resistant to rancidity.

These characteristics make saturated fats the least affected by heat and make them your best choice when it comes to braising, pan frying, baking, roasting and even sautéing.

All foods contain saturated fats.

Animal sources:

- Butter and ghee (clarified butter). Choose those from grass fed, pasture raised cows

- Lard (fat coming from pork)

- Tallow (fat coming from beef)

- Other fats saved from roasting chicken, duck, or goose

- The visible fat on red meat, and under the skin on poultry and fish.

Vegetable sources:

- Coconut oil/butter

- Palm kernel oil/butter

- Cacao butter.

What Is MCT oil?

Medium Chain Triglycerides or MCT are, as the name implies, fatty acids that are of medium length. Fatty acids can be classified based on the number of carbon atoms that makes their chains into short, medium and long chains.

Short chain fatty acids (SCFA) have less than 6 carbon atoms and are absorbed directly into the portal circulation; they don't require bile salts for emulsification and absorption.

Medium chain fatty acids (MCFA) or medium chain triglycerides (MCT) range from 6 carbon to 12 carbon atoms.

Long chain fatty acids (LCFA) have carbon atoms over 12. We will talk later about long chain polyunsaturated fatty acids, omega-6 and-3 (they are C18), and the DHA and EPA, which are C:20.

LCFA require bile for absorption, as well as carnitine to enter the mitochondria and to get oxidized into ketone bodies. It is a much lengthier process.

What's special about MCT?[19]

- they don't require bile salts for absorption (easier for people with sluggish gallbladder function);

- they cross the mitochondrial membrane without the need of carnitine;

- they are rapidly oxidized for energy via beta oxidation; and

- they produce ketone bodies.

One of the best natural, whole food sources of MCT is coconut oil.

If you choose to purchase the MCT oil, look for one that lists all four medium chain fatty acids, as well as the percentage of each one of them. A good one provides Caprylic acid (C8:0) in the greatest concentration (above 50%), as this is the best ketone generating fatty acid with the least undesirable gut irritating effect. There are companies that sell only the isolated Caprylic acid.

When you first add MCT oil to your diet, start with a teaspoon and slowly increase to one tablespoon or more to avoid gastric distress and loose stools.

If your goal is to stick with whole foods, MCT is a refined product, so coconut oil will be the best choice.

> All fats found in nature have some degree of saturation; however, cholesterol is only found in animal foods.
>
> Vegetable fats can be saturated, but are always free of cholesterol.
>
> Even the fats that are classified as saturated fats are not 100% made of SF. They are a mix of mono, poly and saturated fats.

Unsaturated Fatty Acids.

These are classified as poly- and monounsaturated, also known as PUFA and MUFA. Polyunsaturated fats lack many hydrogen atoms on their long carbon chain, which makes them very unstable and easily denatured by oxygen, heat and light. In nature, we find PUFAs in both animal as well as plant foods. They are the essential fatty acids omega-6 (gamma linolenic acid GLA) and omega-3 (alpha linoleic acid ALA).

Plant Sources of Omega-3 Fats:

- Vegetable oils: canola oil

- Seed oils: flax, hemp, chia seeds

- Nut oils: walnuts, almonds

Plant Sources of Omega-6 Fats:

- Vegetable oils: corn, soybean oil, peanut

- Seed oils: sunflower, safflower, pumpkin, sesame, grape

- Nut oils: brazil, macadamia, almond

> *All nuts and seeds contain a mix of omega-6 and omega-3, with more omega-6 than -3. The exception to this is flax seeds, which have more omega-3 than -6 fats.*
>
> *It is better to eat whole nuts and seeds than to consume their extracted oil, as their oils are industry-made oils.*

Animal Sources of PUFAs: EPA (eicosapentaenoic acid) and DHA (docosahexaenoic acid) are the long chain, polyunsaturated fatty acids, the active components of the anti-inflammatory eicosanoid production. The best source of these long chain omega-3 fats are those of marine origin (fatty fish), followed by grass fed, pasture raised animals. Grass-fed land animals have a good fatty acid composition, with a favorable ratio of the omega-6 to omega-3 essential fats.

However, the best food sources for the anti-inflammatory fats are cold water fish such as:

- sardines, mackerel, herring, anchovy, salmon and trout.

The plant sources of omega-3 (ALA), such as those found in flax oil, hemp and chia seeds, still need to be converted in the body into the active forms of DHA and EPA. The conversion rate, however, is low. So, it's best if one acquires the DHA and EPA directly from the sources mentioned above or in a form of high quality fish oil supplement.

How Do You Recognize PUFAs?

- are liquid at room temperature, in the refrigerator and in the freezer;
- are highly affected by heat, oxygen and light; and
- they degrade into highly toxic oxidation products when heated.

Monounsaturated Fatty Acids or MUFA.

In this class, we have two fats:

- omega-9

- omega-7

These fats are a little more saturated (with hydrogen) than the PUFAs, but less than the saturated fats. They only have one double bond or 2 carbon atoms that are not fully saturated with hydrogen (hence the name; mono=one). Because of this, they are more stable, resistant to oxidation and heat damage than the PUFAs, but less stable than the saturated fats. They fall somewhere in the middle.

Omega-9 monounsaturated fat or oleic acid is the most "popular" one with the most health claims (cardio protective benefits) attached to its name.

Food Sources of MUFAs:

- olive oil; and

- almonds, avocados, pecans, cashews, filberts and macadamia nuts.

Animal foods also contain MUFAs, but the main source of mono fats are plant foods.

How Do You Recognize MUFAs?

- They are liquid at room temperature, and become cloudy, thick and clumpy when refrigerated.

Kitchen Tips:

- A good hemp or flax seed oil will be sold in a dark bottle in the refrigerator section of a supermarket.
- It is best to store those oils in the freezer or refrigerator and to use them only on cold dishes.

Regarding vegetable oils (e.g. canola, soybean, corn, peanut): I do not recommend using them at all.

Fats In The Kitchen At a Glance

Best Fats For Cooking	Best Fats For Cold Dishes	Best Fats To Avoid
Coconut oil, butter, ghee (from grass-fed cows) Any animal fat rendered from cooking	Olive oil Flax and hemp seed oils Nuts, seeds and their butters	Canola, corn, soybean, peanut oils All margarines All hydrogenated and partially hydrogenated fats

Kitchen Fun Facts:

When you refrigerate olive oil, it gets thick and forms white clouds. When you turn the bottle upside down, it doesn't run out anymore, but is not completely solid either. If you shake the bottle really hard, it comes out in clumps.

This is a good test to perform to see if you are truly buying a good quality olive oil. If it doesn't get thick and cloudy within 24-48 hours, it is probably a blend that has a great proportion of polyunsaturated vegetable oil added to it.

A good olive oil will be sold in a dark glass bottle, and be labeled extra virgin and cold-pressed.

My recommendation is to use those fats on cold meals (salads and green shakes) or low heat dishes, such as adding them to steamed vegetables.

Store them in dark bottles, inside the cabinet, away from direct light and heat exposure.

My philosophy around olive oil: *"if you pay extra for a cold-pressed, extra virgin olive oil, just keep it that way!"*

Ketones and Ketosis.

I will now switch gears and talk about ketones as the byproduct of a fat burning metabolism.

I introduced ketones previously in the book; in fact more than one time. Unfortunately they have a bad rep.

Why? They were discovered for the first time in the urine of uncontrolled type I diabetics. The phenomenon is known as diabetic ketoacidosis (DKA). It is, indeed, a very dangerous metabolic state, which, if not addressed, can be fatal. It's important to mention here that the reason a person will get in DKA is a lack of insulin, when the pancreas completely loses its insulin secretion function, with excess glucagon secretion, which stimulates overproduction of glucose by the liver (severe hyperglycemia) and accelerated fat burning (severe ketonemia). In diabetic ketoacidosis, we see extremely elevated levels of blood glucose (over 250 mg/dl), along with high blood ketone bodies (over 15-25 mM).[50]

When an individual with a working pancreas, able to maintain normal homeostatic insulin levels, follows a low carb high fat meal plan, they will enter the state of nutritional ketosis (NK). In NK we usually see blood sugar levels below 100 mg/dl, and blood ketones ranging from 0-5 mM. Rarely, they reach 7 or 8 mM when the person follows a prolonged fast. This is defined as starvation ketosis (SK).

It is interesting to mention that even when the blood glucose drops to levels that would be considered hypoglycemic (less than 70 mg/dl), the person will not have the symptoms associated with low blood sugar (shaky, sweaty, and weak), as the ketone bodies fuel the most critical organ: the brain. The brain, at this point, can easily use ketone bodies as its main fuel; hence, it doesn't send emergency signals to the body.

Ketosis Calcification	Ketone Levels mM
No Ketosis	<0.2
Nutritional Ketosis (NK) & Post Exercise Ketosis (EK)	0.5-5
Starvation Ketosis (SK)	5-8
Diabetic Ketoacidosis (DKA)	>10

As you can see, the levels of ketone bodies in nutritional ketosis and even in starvation ketosis are significantly lower than in diabetic ketoacidosis. Comparing those two metabolic states and saying that they are the same is like saying that a summer shower is the same as a hurricane, as they both bring water and wind. I'm sure you'll agree with me that is not the same thing. I live in Florida, and I can tell you hurricanes are no summer showers, despite the fact that both have rain and wind.

> *Normal homeostatic levels of insulin mean the pancreas is able to secrete insulin, just enough to stop the liver from releasing too much glucose (via glycogenolysis or gluconeogenesis) when there is enough glucose in the blood for the organs that rely 100% on it for their function. It's about the fine communication between the insulin and the liver.*

Now that we understand what nutritional ketosis is and that it is safe and very different than DKA, let's look at the ketone bodies and how we can test them.

There are three ketone bodies produced: beta-hydroxybutyrate (B-OHB), acetoacetate and acetone.

There is more than one way to test their presence. Some ways are more accurate than others.

Blood test:

The golden standard is to measure the blood levels of B-OHB. Two drawbacks of this are the cost and the pricking of your fingers.

Urine test:

At first, when you just start this dietary change and your body is in the adaptation phase, you can go by checking your urine with a deep stick for acetoacetate. However, this method is unreliable, as the amount excreted by the kidneys varies greatly independent of ketone levels in the blood and their use by the brain, and the rest of the body, as a source of energy.

Breath test:

This is a non-invasive method, which measures acetone concentration in the breath. Acetoacetate is enzymatically converted to acetone and is eliminated through breath. When people are in ketosis, they can have a fruity breath, due to exhaling acetone. Nowadays, there are several breath ketone meters on the market, and the cost is becoming more affordable. Breath measurements of acetone seem to correlate well with the blood readings of beta-hydroxybutyrate. They require a larger initial investment, but over time, they are a less costly method and are non-invasive.

Ketone's Roles Beyond Fuel.

When researchers first started to look at ketones and their role for us, they thought of them as fat burning metabolites responsible for providing energy to the brain in the absence of glucose. We are now starting to discover a multitude of health benefits ketone bodies play, from drug resistant seizure control, to potent anti-inflammatory agents, epigenetic gene modulation, improvement of cognitive function, anxiety control, reduction of radiation effects on the body (application to space center programs), appetite suppression, cancer growth suppression (indirectly, by starving the cancer, as cancerous cells can't use ketones as energy), activation of mitochondrial function, and shifting white fat to behave more like brown fat. Currently, many studies looking at ketones applications are being done, both on rats and humans. A great website to visit to learn more about the latest on ketones and nutritional ketosis is ketonutrition.org.

As time passes, we will know more about the importance of these metabolites for us that go far beyond energy. For now, let us take maximum advantage of what we already know and allow ketone bodies to help us reverse chronic degenerative and metabolic diseases, reduce inflammation, and power up our brains and bodies to live better, healthier, happier lives.

This concludes the knowledge base on Macronutrients that make the foundation of our food.

In Conclusion.

1. Choose whole foods over processed packaged, industrialized foods.

2. Keep in mind: not all carbs are created equal. If your goal is to lose weight, manage or prevent diabetes, reverse metabolic disorders, improve your energy (mental and physical), break free from food cravings, prevent premature aging, reduce inflammation, live pain free, and heal your gut so you can heal your body, then insulinogenic carbohydrates are not your friend.

3. Make greens and non-starchy vegetables your main source of carbohydrates and fiber.

4. Protein is vital and essential. Keep protein at low to moderate levels and you will support your body to heal, rebuild and stay strong.

5. Make Peace with FAT. Remember: not all fats are created equal. Choose natural fats over industrialized, man-made fats.

At A Glance: A Very Simple Shopping List!
For the complete one, check out the next section Now That You Know, What Do You Do!

☐ Fresh leafy greens and non-starchy vegetables

☐ Fresh eggs from pasture raised chickens

☐ Fresh or frozen meats and fish (not smoked or canned)

☐ Shellfish

☐ Cheese, preferably from grass fed cows

☐ Raw nuts and seeds

☐ Organic cream, butter, ghee, preferably from grass fed cows

☐ Lard, beef tallow, and other animal fats rendered from cooking

☐ Olive oil, coconut oil, cacao butter

☐ Avocado

☐ Garlic, Celtic Sea Salt or Himalayan Crystal Salt

☐ Spices and herbs

☐ Berries and other low glycemic fruits according to your unique carbohydrate tolerance

PART 4: FASTING 101

Adding fasting to the low carb, high fat eating style is 10Xing your results. In this section, we'll see why that is.

I'd like to ask you first: What does fasting means to you? What kind of emotions does it bring up? How do you look at the possibility of abstaining from food?

Pause for a moment and give yourself an answer to those questions.

In my experience, bringing up the word "fasting" is like saying the F word. Seriously! It is so ingrained in people's minds that they need to eat every 2-3 hours that if you tell them to fast they think you're cursing them or you're passing the death sentence upon them.

Do you feel that way, too?

Whether you do or not, I think this section will help you look at fasting with different eyes. You'll begin to love the two F words: Fast and Fat!

Steps In Health Transformation

Do not panic! You don't have to do anything you are not ready to do. Remember, first is the mindset, then the action. The first step in a health transformation is becoming aware of the need to change. The second is having the knowledge that strengthens the new belief. The third comes with embedding the new beliefs until they became your new reality: e.g. "Fasting is good for me." "It's ok to skip a meal or two." "Fasting is healing." The fourth is you take action based on knowledge and from a place of strong belief.

Fasting is as old as human history! Whether it was imposed on us by nature and the environment we lived in (as it was for the caveman), or intended, as we see in many forms of religion, it is safe to say that humans have always fasted.

Food for thought

In the past 50 years or so, fasting lost its popularity. We were advised by the experts to eat every 2-3 hours, as that somehow would help us lose weight. Our lifestyle became more sedentary, as many human energy saving devices showed up in our existence, such as drive thrus, escalators, elevators, remote controls, and so on. Food become abundant and of poor quality.

We created the perfect nutrition and lifestyle storm. 50 years later, we collect the results in the form of more diabetes and prediabetes, more overweight people and obesity, more cardiovascular disease, more cancer, and more chronic diseases than ever before in human history.

I say it's time to change that. It's a good time to eat less often, less food, real food, and real fats; and to spend more time outdoors, in nature, engaged in fun activities with family and friends.

By the strictest definition, fasting is *"abstinence from all food."* However, there are many modified fasts, which are good variations of the strict water fast. Below I'm listing the most commonly used forms of fast:

- Water fast. Total restriction from food with water only allowed.

- Fat fast. The person consumes fat, but refrains from the other two macronutrients. As so fat mimics fasting or starvation. Fat fast provides the body with calories, without interfering with the energy metabolism hormones. I find for most people it's easier to do a fat fast, at least when they are new to the fasting practice. One way to do a fat fast is to drink a hot coffee or tea with fat added to it. A popular example is the bullet-proof coffee made of French press or espresso coffee, grass fed butter and MCT oil.

- Modified liquid fast. Allows meat/bone stock, fermented beverages, such as the brine from lacto-fermented vegetables or sauerkraut juice, juiced green vegetables (e.g. cabbage, cucumbers, parsley, cilantro), ginger and turmeric roots, lemon juice or apple cider vinegar, and herbal teas.

A Few Reasons to Consider Fasting.

Fasting is the best way to overcome emotional attachment to food, and to address physical and mental stagnation, which can manifest as apathy, fatigue, depression and chronic degenerative conditions. It's a great way to purify the body after times of feasting, before changing seasons or major life events, or even before trying a new way of eating. Fasting is used for spiritual reasons; meditation and clarity; to enhance mental awareness, sleep and dreams; to optimize brain function; longevity; and to support healthy aging[26].

Fasting is the fastest way to jumpstart and to maintain a fat burning metabolism, and to enter the nutritional ketosis zone. It turns on genes that help cells survive by reducing global inflammation. Calorie Restriction (CR) as a result of fasting may improve nerve function, and support memory and cognition. CR below Basal Metabolic Rate (BMR) allows the brain to make new neurons (by decreasing free radicals), enhances the ability to generate ATP for energy, and increases the number of mitochondria.

It turns out that the many health benefits of fasting can be attributed to the suppressing effect it has on the mTOR pathway—which makes the body enter "self-eating" mode—as well as, to a large degree, to the buildup of ketone bodies to therapeutic levels, ranging from 0.5-5, and even up to 7 mM. Due to the lowering effect fasting has on insulin and blood sugar, it helps reverse insulin resistance and associated metabolic disorders[27].

During fasting, vital survival adaptive mechanisms are turned on. Your brain becomes more alert; you think more clearly, are sharper and are able to make fast decisions. Ketones seem to promote changes in structure and function of neurons, and increase the number of mitochondria. The gene that's responsible for the synthesis of brain derived neurotrophic factor (BDNF) is activated as well. BDNF is a protein that protects neurons and plays a role in creating new neurons. It acts like a growth hormone for neurons and is vital for thinking, learning and a higher level of brain function[28]. It makes sense for this to happen. Our ancestors went through many fasts, some longer and some shorter. If, while fasting, we couldn't effectively use our brains, we wouldn't be here as a species. In the absence of food, the brain creates new and stronger neuronal connections (BDNF being responsible for this), so we can think better and faster; hence, we can find and catch our next meal.

In this state of emergency (fasting), the body becomes "wiser" with regards to the way it operates, to what tissues it allocates more fuel, and how it generates fuel.

How does the body maintain normal blood glucose during a fast?

The liver produces glucose via gluconeogenesis. To do that, it uses amino acid and the glycerol bone of fatty acids. The glycerol bone is supplied by fatty acids metabolism. In other words, when the fat is burned for fuel it releases the glycerol bone. The glycerol is then used to make glucose along with the glucogenic amino acids.

What about the amino acids? Where do they come from in the absence of food (if we fast)?

During prolonged fasting (over 72 hours), the body begins to use as a substrate to make glucose its own "spare" amino acids, such as those that would be used to make digestive enzymes (there is nothing to digest, so there is no need to make those) or those that would be used to make sex hormones (who wants to reproduce in the middle of a crisis?). It also searches for damaged cells, denatured DNA, and cancerous cells, and uses them as substrate to make glucose.

This is part of the deep cellular cleanse (detox) initiated by the suppression of mTOR.

What happens metabolically during fasting?

When we eat, we store energy.

First, we fill up the small glycogen tanks (liver and muscles), about 2000 calories, then we fill up the large fat reservoir, over 40,000 calories.

When we don't eat, and I'm not talking about 3 hours in between meals, the body uses up most of the liver glycogen (glycogenolysis) to supply glucose for the body. This can take up to 48 hours, depending on a person's age and activity level.

When the glycogen tank is empty, or it gets alarmingly low, the body shifts to burning fat as fuel and produces ketone bodies (liver beta oxidation).

At the same time, the liver turns on alternative pathways to produce glucose and it maintains normal glycemia (gluconeogenesis).

Therefore,

- there is enough glucose to supply energy for the cells that rely on it exclusively (e.g. red blood cells, retina of the eye and the liver itself);

- ketones become the preferred fuel for the brain, the "emergency" organ; and

- the rest of the body uses a mix of ketones and fatty acids.

The body has this inner wisdom and built in survival mechanism. When it comes to critical times, it stops wasting energy with the organs that don't serve a vital role or with the functions that are not prime real estate. It is all so beautifully and perfectly orchestrated to assure our survival, and to keep us healthy.

If the body gets into a self-cleaning mode when we don't eat—and that is good for healing and longevity—why are we advised to eat every 2-3 hours? How is that benefiting us? In fact, calorie restriction studies done on rats and monkeys prove the less they eat the longer they live and vice versa. Some studies even report that fasting inhibits the growth of spontaneous cancers[38].

Eating and converting food into energy generate free radicals, or oxidative damage. When food is converted to energy (inside the mitochondria) during the process of energy generation (in the form of ATP-adenosine triphosphate), free radicals (reactive oxygen species ROS) are produced. Of all three macronutrients, carbohydrates are the most "polluting" fuel. When glucose is burned to produce ATP (energy), it generates more free radicals than the fat does[19]. This is another reason to eat less food in general and less carbohydrates in particular. Fasting and a low carb, high fat eating style make a good partnership, not only when it comes to metabolic health and inflammation but with regards to oxidative damage as well.

In summary, when we abstain from food, the body:

- eats out damaged cellular parts and gets rid of cellular junk (detox at the cellular level)—a process controlled by the mTOR pathway.

- starts burning fat, as food energy is not available and generates ketones, which then exert many health benefits aside from brain fuel.

- strengthens and protects the mitochondria.

- insulin levels drop and remain low.

- inflammation is reduced and less reactive oxygen species are produced (aka. free radicals).

This creates an overall healing environment at the cellular level.

While you can't fast forever, you can follow a low-carb, high-fat, moderate protein diet, and when you combine it with fasting, you 10X your results.

> *Keep in mind that, when it comes to healing with foods or preventing disease with foods, what you eat, how much you eat and how often you eat are all important.*

The longest recorded water fast is held by a 27-year-old young man. In 1973, a study reported that this young man went for a total of 382 days with no food; only water, vitamins and minerals. Yes, that's how much energy this person had stored over the years inside his adipose tissues. He had enough energy to fuel his body for over a year! He started at a weight of 456 lbs. and lost 276 lbs. in 382 days. This was, of course, medically supervised[29].

If he could do it for 382 days, don't you think you can do it for 18 or 24 hours? I'm sure you can!

Although there are many ways you can fast, there is no right or wrong way; it's a matter of finding what works best for you. Here are some possibilities:

- Intermittent fast (IF), a compressed eating window (6-8 hours of eating out of 24 hour day)

- 24 hour fast (dinner to dinner, or lunch to lunch)

- 72 hour fast

- Alternate day fasting

- Prolonged fast (7-21 or more days)

Nevertheless, the most healing and therapeutic is the water fast; however, the liquid fasts that allow fat, tea, meat/bone stock and fermented beverages are also beneficial.

Personally, I'm a big fan of daily, intermittent fasting (IF) in the form of a compressed eating window. What that means is if we take the 24 hour day (plus night) and we look at when we eat first and last meals of the day, that is the window of eating. Most people eat from the time they wake up until the time they go to sleep. Let's say that's from 7 am to 9 pm, then that's a total of a 14 hour eating window, with 10 hours of overnight fasting. Fasting compresses the window of eating to 6-8 hours and increases the fasting period to 16-18 hours. This is done daily.

As an example, for me socially, it makes sense to eat my food later in the day, as we all sit down for dinner as a family. So, for the first part of the day, I only drink water and 1, sometimes 2, bulletproof coffees (fat fast). I break my fast anywhere from 2 pm to 5 pm, depending on the day, and I usually stop eating by 8 pm, so my fasting varies from 18 to 21 hours.

For an in depth look at fasting, I recommend reading the book "The Complete Guide to Fasting" by Jason Fung, MD and Jimmy Moore.

Is fasting for everyone? No!

Who should not consider fasting?

- Pregnant and lactating women

- Underweight individuals

- Individuals with adrenal and thyroid dysfunction (take it with caution)

- Individuals on multiple drugs (it can be done under strict medical supervision)

- Type 1 diabetics (can partake, but require direct medical supervision)

What are your thoughts on fasting, after reading this chapter? Are you less scared of it? Is it something you're ready to try?

If you are not, take your time. Read more, learn more, contemplate more; one day you will feel ready and you will do it.

If you are ready, congrats! Go for it. But, nevertheless, make sure to check with your medical doctor before starting any fast and even before adopting this way of eating, especially if you are taking multiple drugs to manage diseases.

It's best to have a team of practitioners that offer you their support and attention. Feel free to offer them a copy of this book to help them understand the way you intend to manage your disease with food, fast and lifestyle.

Now, we can move into the action stage. Next: Now That You Know, What Do You Do!

Awareness And Knowledge At A Glance:

We first looked at what food is, the definition of food and the criteria to use to make wholesome food choices.

Then we looked at the "meaning" of food beyond calories and pleasure. We learned that food is powerful information for your genes, and it can change the script of your inherited genetic material.

We looked at how food controls metabolism by the way it interacts with the hormones that regulate energy production.

We dove into the three main factors that contribute to chronic disease today: hyperinsulinemia and IR, global low grade inflammation and the state of the gut, its microflora.

We reviewed the three macronutrients food provides for us with their sources and main roles in the body, from health to energy.

We concluded that the common dietary change that gives us the most in return revolves around carbohydrates.

We learned how to formulate a therapeutic low carb, moderate protein and high fat eating plan.

Last but not least, we looked at the power of abstaining from food and how that is beneficial to us, from healing to spiritual benefits.

ACTION

PART 5: NOW THAT YOU KNOW, WHAT DO YOU DO!

Now that you know, you are probably asking: what do I do, Mihaela? How do I start this way of eating? What should I expect to feel and when will I start to feel better?

There is no single, straightforward answer to those questions, as each person is unique and responds differently. *"You are the study of one."* I will outline here the approach that works for many, and you can adapt it to your unique lifestyle, life circumstances and health goals.

I designed this part of the book to help you take action; it is more like a workbook. I provide the step-by-step system I use with my private clients. Take it as blueprint or as a guide, and apply it to your unique situation.

There are a few stages you'll need to go through.

The first stage involves your mindset for success. The other ones have to do with getting your body adapted to a new way of eating, and organizing your life so you can follow through.

Keep in mind why you are doing this.

Why are you choosing broccoli over potatoes, kale over rice, or avocado over banana? What is the reason? What is the benefit? What are you getting in return?

Review the knowledge base that was covered in the first part of the book if you are not clear on the why and how. But even more important than the sciencey why, is your personal why!

Why do you want to lose weight? Why do you want to go off prescription drugs? Why do you want to have more energy? And so on. In other words what is your inner, deeper motivating factor? When you are crystal clear about that, the entire process that's outlined here will go relatively smooth.

Step 1. Get very clear about what are you trying to achieve with food (and lifestyle)

Take a journal and write down your life and health goals, or you may use the form below.

Begin with the big picture goals and break them down to today's goals.

10 year goals _____

_____

_____

_____

5 year goals _____

_____

_____

_____

1 year goals _____

_____

_____

_____

6 month goals _____

_____

_____

_____

3 month goals _____

_____

_____

_____

1 month goals _____

_____

_____

_____

1 week goals _____

_____

_____

_____

Today's goals _____

_____

_____

_____

Review these goals daily. Make a daily ritual of goal setting and goal reviewing.

What I often see happening is that people set up big, bold goals; they write them in a journal; and then they put it aside and simply forget about their goals. Life gets busy and nothing changes. You've got to look at your goals daily, and take action daily.

Below, you'll see some examples of goals that either I or some of my clients had. You, of course, will set your own goals. These are just to help you get started.

☐ Weight loss + maintenance. I want to lose 30 pounds by the time I turn 55 and keep it off forever

☐ Blood sugar management. I want to manage good glycemic control through food and lifestyle

☐ Eliminate over the counter or prescription drugs (diabetes, lipid management, pain meds)

☐ Sustained energy from when I wake up until I go to bed at night

☐ Stable moods, feeling in control of my life instead of life controlling me

☐ By next summer be comfortable in a bikini

☐ Run a half marathon for the Autism Foundation

☐ Normalize bowel movements, get rid of bloating, gas, acid reflux

Please complete this step before moving onto the next. Clarity of goals is paramount to your success. You can have more than one goal, but pick no more than 3 to work on at one time; it will reduce feelings of being overwhelmed and increase your success rate. Thus, it will boost your confidence and you'll be able to tackle more after that.

When you set goals, set S.M.A.R.T. goals.

S.M.A.R.T. goals are used in time management and marketing projects, but they can be very well adapted to any goals including personal health and wellness goals.[39]

Let's take an example of a S.M.A.R.T goal:

"In 6 months, I'd like to significantly improve my glycemic control. My doctor told me I'm pre-diabetic and my goal is, when I go for my next 6 month check-up, to have my HbA1C in the normal range. I'd like to have my HbA1C drop from 6.3 to 5.4. I will achieve this through food and lifestyle. To be more precise, I will start the metabolic reset protocol as my dietary strategy."

Specific: Be clear and specific with your goals. What will you do and how will you do it?

e.g. *"I want to improve my glycemic control.... through food and lifestyle. To be more precise, I will start the metabolic reset protocol as my dietary strategy."*

Measurable: You or anyone else looking at your goals should be able to measure progress/outcomes. You need to have tangible evidence that you've accomplished your goal.

e.g. *"I'd like to have my HbA1C drop from 6.3 to 5.4."*

Attainable: The goals you set need to feel a little challenging to you, but, at the same time, you need to be confident that you possess the knowledge, skills, tools, support and ability needed to reach those goals.

In our example, the person needs to know exactly what the metabolic reset protocol is, and what it takes to implement it. He needs to follow a guide or work closely with someone who can coach him through the process.

Result oriented: This means that you are looking at the outcomes of reaching this goal and not at the activities you are engaging in to achieve the goal. In simpler terms, you keep in mind the main benefits associated with reaching your goal. Keep at the top of your mind the big picture while doing the teeny tiny tasks.

In the example, the person will focus on having good glycemic control, losing weight, having more energy, just being a healthy person, and living a stress-free life.

Time bound: The goals need to have a deadline to create a practical sense of urgency and excitement for crossing the finish line.

In the example, this person has six months to reach his goal.

Step 2. Find ways to measure progress and outcomes

The reason I recommend this step is to have a more objective way of measuring. You, me or anyone else should be able to measure the outcomes of the goals you set for yourself. *Ultimately, the best way of measuring progress and outcomes is in how you feel.* However, having some baseline biometric markers that will change over time is a powerful incentive or reassuring factor both for you and for the team of practitioners you'll be working with.

Next, I'll list the biometric markers I use with my private clients.

☐ **Baseline laboratory exams**

In the first part of this book, I explained the laboratory tests that are relevant when it comes to your metabolic health and inflammation. Here, I'm just giving you a list of the most important ones so you can collaborate with your doctor and order them. Some of them will be performed and covered by medical insurance only if you have a family history of diabetes and cardiovascular disease. If you choose to pay out of pocket, you can order all of them.

☐ **Anthropometrics**

Anthropometrics means measuring the size, weight and the proportions of the body.

Waist and hip measurements.

Here it is important to measure your waist and hip circumference, and to calculate your waist to hip ratio. Current guidelines by WHO state that a waist to hip ratio of >0.85 for women and >0.9 for men is indicative of dangerous abdominal obesity and increased risk for developing cardio metabolic diseases. The American Heart Association defines abdominal obesity as a waist circumference >35 inches for women and >45 inches for men.

Pertinent Laboratory Tests

- CBC and CMP (these are usually done routinely)

- Vit D (25 hydroxy Vitamin D)

- HbA1C

- Fasting Insulin

- Fasting BS

- Oral Glucose Tolerance Test and Insulin Response (this is more difficult to obtain, but important if you suspect you are at risk of developing diabetes. In other words, you are in the early pre-diabetic stages and want to proactively take measures to prevent the onset of diabetes)

- Homocysteine

- hs-CRP

- Feritin

- B12

- Lipid particle size tests (NMR LipoProfile Test (developed by Lab-Corp), Lipoprotein Particle Profile (LPP) Test (developed by Spectra-Cell), Cardio IQ Report (offered through Quest Diagnostics)

- Omega-3 Index [this test measures omega-3 fatty acids, DHA and EPA in red blood cells and is used to assess cardiovascular risk. Proposed omega-3 index risk zones are (in percentages of erythrocyte FAs): high risk, <4%; intermediate risk, 4–8%; and low risk, >8% [30]

Weight and body composition.

If you have a scale or another device that measures body composition available, it is a great way to track, not only your total weight, but also your body composition (fat%, water %, fat free muscle mass (FFMM) in pounds or Kg). For the body composition table please refer back to Fat 101, side bar: "White fat and brown fat!"

It is nice to see total weight loss, but knowing how much of that loss is attributed to fat versus lean tissue (muscles) is so much more powerful.

I use a Tanita scale in my practice to measure body composition and to track progress overtime.

☐ **Outfit fitting (if weight loss is one of your goals)**

I believe this is the most fun way to measure your weight and body composition changes. You pick an outfit you love, but is a bit too tight on you (the dream outfit to fit in in, let's say, 3 months). Take some pictures in it and keep putting it on once a month. You'll be able to see it getting bigger and bigger on you, as you are losing weight and changing body size.

☐ **Before and after photos (if weight loss is one of your goals)**

These are also fun. You can take front, back and sideways shots before you start your new food and lifestyle. Then, do it again every 3 or 6 months after that. You choose!

Step 3. Set up your winning environment

Please do not underestimate the power of your environment.

☐ **People, family, friends, accountability partner**

I'm sure you understand the power of support. To be successful, you need to be determined to take action; however, surrounding yourself with people that are doing the same, or, better yet, are already there, can 10X your results.

Keep in mind this quote by motivational speaker Jim Rohn: *"You are the average of the five people you spend most of your time with."* Choose your friends wisely!

☐ **Books and other resources (programs, groups, cookbooks, and health books, such as this one)**

This is pretty self-explanatory. In fact, I'm sure right now you have many health books, plenty of cookbooks and websites you go to for recipes, you belong to many groups, and probably have bought many health, weight loss, detox, etc. programs. There's never a shortage of resources.

What keeps most people stuck is a lack of deep, inner motivation and awareness. That's why one of my main goals for writing this book was to make you aware of the immense power that the food you put in your mouth 3 or more times a day plays in your health; to empower you with knowledge; to help you understand how you can use food to heal; to help set you free of fear and confusion, frustration and being overwhelmed; and to give you the tools you need to take consistent actions so you can see measurable and lasting results.

Note: When you purchased this book, you were granted access to my private "Make Peace With Fat" Community. If you didn't join us there, **go to www.facebook.com/Groups/MakePeaceWithFat and join us** now. That's where I provide daily live support and help leverage even more of what you are learning from this book.

☐ **Coach or mentor**

This is the most important external factor that can 100X your results. The support, guidance and accountability you receive when you work with a qualified coach or mentor are priceless.

☐ **Medical team**

I believe it is extremely important to build a team of practitioners that will help you go through this healing journey. This should include a medical doctor and his staff that understand the role food plays in health and healing—it is important that they are familiar with the metabolic and gut reset therapies. Your job is to interview as many doctors as it takes until you find the one that you like and feel that you can form a partnership with. He or she will help you order the pertinent labs, monitor your progress and help manage your drug therapy, should you be taking any.

For a list of practitioners that are using metabolic therapies in their practice check: https://www.ketonutrition.org/resources.

For practitioners specialized in gut healing protocols check: http://www.gaps.me/find-a-gaps-practitioner.php.

Step 4. Get your kitchen and pantry ready

Finally, we are making our way to the kitchen. Yes, it's time to focus on getting your kitchen ready, as well as revamping your refrigerator and pantry. Learn how to shop in the grocery store; how to read the food labels, should you choose to buy packaged foods; and, finally, how to locate local farmer's markets, get to know the farmers, make connections with them and let them become the main food provider for you and your family.

Kitchen tools

When it comes to kitchen tools, please take into consideration the materials your cooking and storing dishes are made of. I invite you to walk through all your cabinets and gather all of the plastic, aluminum, Teflon, and other reactive material that potentially can contribute to the toxic load in your life and add more inflammation. Inflammation is caused by any type of injury, including from your cookware. Use cookware and storage dishes made of stainless steel, glass or ceramic. Please see the Kitchen Tools Resource Guide for details.

Kitchen Tools Resource Guide:

- ☐ Kitchen scale (preferably an electronic one)
- ☐ Blender:
    - o large enough (2L/quart container)
    - o glass or BPA, PVC free container
    - o high performance
- ☐ Food processor:
    - o 4-9 cup container
    - o BPA, PVC free container
- ☐ Steamer:
    - o stainless steel and large enough 4-6 quarts base container
- ☐ Salad bowls:
    - o stainless steel
    - o glass or ceramic (must be careful, as it can break and shatter-leads to injuries)
    - o wood or bamboo
- ☐ Sautéing pan:
    - o stainless steel (preferably surgical grade)
- ☐ Slow cooker:
    - o 6-8 quarts
- ☐ Baking pans:
    - o ceramic or glass
- ☐ Soup pot:
    - o stainless steel (preferably surgical grade)
    - o about 8 quarts
- ☐ Fine sieve
- ☐ Cutting boards:
    - o bamboo or wood
    - o large and small
- ☐ Knifes:
    - o 1 or 2 stainless steel or ceramic knives
    - o chef's knife and paring knife
- ☐ Vegetable spinner:
    - o large enough, about 2-5 quarts
- ☐ Canning jars:
    - o many sizes for many purposes (pickling, storing, etc.)

Where to get all these?

- o Amazon, or local stores like Target or Home Goods

Pantry + refrigerator cleanup and restocking

This is an important step and it's a very emotionally charged one. You will have a lot of resistance when it comes to actually doing this step. If you find yourself pushing it off or procrastinating, then hire someone to do it for you. Give them the criteria to use for the cleanup, provide them with a big trash bag or boxes, so they can pack away the no longer acceptable food items. You may choose to donate them to a local food bank or to simply trash them.

It's up to you, but the pantry and refrigerator need to be cleaned and room needs to be made for the whole, healing foods that are now making their way into your life.

Criteria for cleaning up the pantry and for future shopping of packaged food.

You will be reading the ingredients list and eliminating the foods that come with any of the following:

1. **Sugar.** (Refer to the many names of sugar in the Carbohydrates 101 section of the book if you are not sure what those are.)

2. **Artificial sweeteners.** A few examples would be Saccharin, Acesulfame K, Sucralose (Splenda®), and Aspartame (NutraSweet®, Equal®).

3. **Food colorings, preservatives and flavorings.** There are too many to list here, but think names you can't pronounce or read easily. Some examples of food color additives are: FD&C Blue Nos. 1 and 2, FD&C Green No. 3, FD&C Red Nos. 3 and 40, FD&C Yellow Nos. 5 and 6, Orange B, Citrus Red No. 2, annatto extract, beta-carotene, grape skin extract, cochineal extract or carmine, paprika oleoresin, and caramel color.

Note: Certain color additives are "exempt," meaning they are not required to be declared by name on labels, but may be declared simply as colorings or color added). For a complete list check out www.fda.gov/food/ingredientspackgingla-beling/. [31]

4. **Vegetable oils, hydrogenated and partially hydrogenated oils.** For a refresher about vegetable oils and their contribution to inflammation and ill health, refer to the "FATS 101" section. Some examples are soybean oil, corn oil, canola oil, peanut oil and hydrogenated soybean oil.

5. **Alcohol.** It's best to eliminate it all, but if you choose to keep any, make it "on the rocks" or dry wine. Refer to the alcohol section found under Carbohydrates 101 for more details about this.

By following the above criteria, you are eliminating 80-90% of all packaged foods. Use the same criteria for when you go shopping as well. You will be surprised to find out how many foods like sausages, mustards, dressings and ketchups are loaded with one or more of the above ingredients. Similarly, baked goods, from bread to cookies and cakes, chips, pretzels, etc., aside from being made of grains and starches, contain these items.

Hydration beverages.

When it comes to beverages, the best beverage of all is water. Good pure water.

Choose spring water if possible; if not, invest in a good water filtration system. If you wish to flavor your water, you can add to it essential oils, sliced cucumbers, strawberries, lemon, ginger or fresh mint leaves. Any fresh vegetables, fruit or herbs will work as well.

Take fresh water in a 2 quart glass jar, add to it slices of the vegetable or fruit you wish, and keep it in the refrigerator overnight. The next day you will have a refreshing, healthy, naturally flavored water.

What should you drink if you exercise and sweat a lot? Is the answer Gatorade®?

If you sweat a lot, add salt to your water. We'll talk more about salt later, but for now let's focus on hydration.

Do this test the next time you sweat: lick your skin on your arm. What do you taste? Salt, right? That tells you exactly what you lose mostly through sweat. You lose sodium, so adding salt to your water helps you rehydrate your body, replenish lost sodium and reinvigorates you. You don't need sugar and artificial colorings from Gatorade®. Save the money and buy real food.

Another great post-exercise beverage you can have is a good, old fashioned, homemade chicken stock salted with Celtic sea salt or Himalayan Crystal salt. This is not only a good source of amino acids (needed for muscle recovery), but also of potassium, and other minerals that leach into the stock/broth from the bones and the meat.

You can also drink the brine from lacto-fermented vegetables or sauerkraut juice.

Now, we're talking about rehydrating your body, and healing with foods all at the same time.

If you are an athlete and you can "afford more carbohydrates," then coconut water during and post-exercise is the best sports drink.

No fruit juices please. Even if you make them fresh from organic fruits, they have too much sugar that is too easily absorbed. The glucose from juice spikes insulin and the fructose turns rapidly into fat in your liver. Just eat the whole fruit with its skin. Go for berries, as they have more fiber and the pigments in berries are strong antioxidants. Refer to the resources section, for a table with different berries and their macronutrient breakdown.

Help to transition from soda to water. Kombucha – it is a fermented drink, so it helps inoculate your gut with friendly microbes. It's carbonated, kind of like soda, not as sweet, but sweet enough to do the trick. It has some residual sugar and, eventually, you will need to figure out how to make it fit your daily "carb bank," or stop drinking it. For the transition phase, you don't need to worry about it; it's a great crutch you can use as needed.

Foods that come in jars or other packages.

Below you'll find the shopping list of foods that although are not processed come in jars, bottles, or other packages, and you will buy on a regular basis. They are staple foods.

As you become more acquainted with this way of eating, and learn how to read food labels and what ingredients to look for, you will come across other packaged foods that are made of whole foods ingredients, are low carb, and contain natural fat, which you will be able to enjoy.

Packaged Foods Shopping List

☐ Condiments, seaweed, spices, cacao powder, salt, pepper

☐ Fats: butter, ghee, sour cream, heavy cream, coconut oil, olive oil, cacao butter

☐ Raw nuts and seeds, and their butters

☐ Olives

☐ Proteins: eggs, cheese, sardines, and other wild caught fish (look for BPA free cans)

☐ Apple cider vinegar

☐ Mustard

☐ Ferments: sauerkraut, lacto fermented cucumbers, kimchi, kombucha

☐ Other foods: coconut wraps, RX-Bar, LaraBar, Kelp noodles, Miracle noodles, Primal Kitchen Mayonnaise, dark chocolate (Alter Eco Super Blackout 90% cacao), meat sticks

Don't dread this step. Think how much it will help you not to have the trigger foods around you. You can make this a one week goal and break it into daily goals, so it gets done within the time frame you choose. Give yourself a deadline and go complete this step.

Please don't skip this step unless you're already eating whole foods. Your overall success really depends on what foods you have available in the house for when you need to cook in a hurry, you have cravings or you are super hungry. Having foods available that support your goals makes it 10X easier to stick to the plan.

"Out of sight out of mind" works well, especially when it comes to trigger foods—you know the ones that "call your name and attention" every time you are happy, sad, anxious, bored, etc. Make it part of your winning environment to keep in the house only foods that support you, and not those that sabotage your success.

At the completion of this step (getting your kitchen and pantry ready), you should be eating mostly whole foods. At this stage, you are eating a diet free of added sugar, food additives and vegetable oils. This is the first step in reducing inflammation and even dropping a few pounds—depending on your starting point, how processed your diet was and how often you drank beverages other than water.

How long will it take you to complete this step is entirely up to you. I suggest no more than 1 week, but, again, this is your health journey. You are in the driver's seat. You are making the decisions.

Next, let me introduce the two healing with foods protocols:

☐ The metabolic reset protocol (MRP)

☐ The gut reset protocol (GRP)

The metabolic reset protocol encompasses two levels of intervention and is achieved by adjusting the macronutrient ratios of the whole foods you eat. This is a hormonal and intracellular food "intervention."

MRP at a glance:

The hormonal intervention aims to lower insulin and to re-sensitize the body to its action (reverse or reduce insulin resistance). This is accomplished mainly through carbohydrate restriction, mainly elimination of all sugar, grains, legumes and starches, and through fasting. As a result, global low grade inflammation is also reduced.

The intracellular intervention aims to power-up mitochondrial function. This is mainly achieved through the combined forces of carbohydrate restriction and simultaneous increase in fat consumption. Fasting 10Xs this effect.

It is under these circumstances when the body begins to favor fat burning—ketone bodies are produced and they exert their "magic" power on the mitochondria. We see more and better functioning mitochondria. They become more effective at converting fat to ketones; the whole energy production goes up. Less free radicals are produced by burning cleaner fuel and global low grade inflammation is reduced as well.

The gut reset protocol also includes two levels of intervention: cellular and microbial. The cellular approach aims to support optimal enterocyte function for proper nutrition absorption, while the microbial intervention focuses on rebalancing the gut flora—the main controller of gut health and overall health.

GRP at a glance:

Restoring the enterocytes function and gut integrity involves the removal of all processed foods, sugar, grains, legumes and starches.

As you can see, there is a nice overlap with the metabolic reset plan.

Aside from the elimination, GRP adds nourishing foods specific to rebuilding the enterocytes (amino acids and fats provided by animal foods—mainly joints, bones and bone marrow, fat, organ meats).

Finally, rebalancing of the gut flora is mainly done by the addition of fermented foods, as well as therapeutic strength probiotics.

You may be asking, *"When will I use one protocol over the other?" "Should I use both?" "If I need to use both, which one should I start with or should I combine them?"*

The good thing about the two protocols is that they greatly overlap and, in fact, they complement each other. They both eliminate insulinogenic carbohydrates. While MRP focuses on the macronutrient ratios, the gut protocol emphasizes the nutrient density of foods with a focus on gut rebuilding.

Merging the two is, by far, more powerful than doing one over the other. However, since not everyone needs to be on a strict nutritional ketosis all the time, I will present them separately.

If you were to combine them, I suggest adding the more nourishing gut foods (meat/bone stock, organ meats) and the fermented foods to the metabolic reset protocol (MRP), and stay on the adaptation phase for as long as you feel you are getting results. I spent 3 full years on that phase.

When should you use the metabolic reset protocol (most of these are related to insulin resistance, but not all)? If you have any of the below conditions or a family history, you may want to start with the MRP.

- ☐ Obesity, overweight

- ☐ Prediabetes or diabetes

- ☐ Metabolic syndrome

☐ Fatty liver

☐ Polycystic ovarian syndrome (PCOS)

☐ Dyslipidemia

☐ Hypertension

☐ Sleep apnea

☐ Gastroesophageal reflux disease (GERD)

☐ Drug-resistant seizures

☐ Endurance performance

The gut reset protocol is to be used primarily by people that suffer from:

☐ Inflammatory gut diseases such as irritable bowel syndrome (IBS), inflammatory bowel disease (IBD), colitis, ulcerative colitis (UC)

☐ Acid reflux, GERD, gas, bloating, diarrhea, constipation

☐ Food sensitivities

☐ Migraine headaches

☐ Arthritis

☐ Anxiety, depression and other mood disorders

☐ Autoimmune disease [lupus, rheumatoid arthritis (RA), Crohn's disease, Hashimoto's thyroiditis, multiple sclerosis (MS)]

If you happen to fit into both categories, then it is best to prioritize your health goals and see which one of your health problems requires immediate attention, and that's how you know which protocol to begin with.

Again, they overlap greatly. However, the MRP puts a greater emphasis on the macronutrient ratios and hitting certain target numbers for carbohydrates, proteins and fats, while the GRP is more liberal when it comes to macronutrient ratios. The main objective of GRP is to eliminate the "gut-damaging foods," and puts a greater emphasis on supplying the healing elements that rebuild the gut lining and rebalance the gut microflora. Please keep in mind food quality and nutrient density are more important than food quantity. As an example, when you choose your protein, it is best to get the most nutrient dense animal protein which is found in organ meats of grass fed animals (e.g. liver, not in the expensive filet mignon).

Now, let's take them one at a time.

PART 5.1:
THE METABOLIC RESET PROTOCOL (MRP)

Starting on the metabolic reset journey is like going up a mountain, you get tired and you want to quit before you reach the summit; but when you look back, you realize you are closer to the summit than to the base of the mountain. So, you keep climbing! Once you reach the summit, you feel amazing. You feel like you are on top of the world. From there, you look down on the other side; the valley you are heading towards is just amazing, like a paradise.

You begin your descent and, once on the other side, you feel like you are living your dream life; a life free of uncontrollable hunger and food cravings. For the first time, food doesn't rule your life; it doesn't take over your entire brain space. You begin to do the things you love and could only dream of doing. Your energy is surging, your health improves by the day, you take fewer drugs or perhaps no drugs at all, your body is not aching—in fact, you feel good in your body. You are happier, more confident and life becomes amazing again. You are so glad you climbed that mountain and crossed over it.

Let's climb this mountain together, shall we?

Phase 1: Initiation and adaptation

In this phase, your goal is to jumpstart the fat burning metabolism to get your body to shift from a glucose-based fuel to a fat-based fuel where ketone bodies are easily produced and used as an energy source.

This is the equivalent of climbing the mountain in our beginning story. It can take anywhere from 3 to 5 or even more weeks, depending on your unique body. But 3-4 weeks is what it takes for most people.

To keep this transition as simple as possible for the first 3 weeks, just focus on eliminating the foods that are high in insulinogenic carbohydrates. Refer to the complete shopping list to see exactly what you will be eating.

> *In this phase, focus on what you eat and do not think about the macronutrient ratios. Just pay attention to satiety. Eat to fullness and satisfaction.*

These are the foods you will be eliminating:

- ☐ Sugar and anything that contains sugar

- ☐ Grains and anything made of grains

- ☐ Starchy vegetables

- ☐ Legumes

- ☐ Milk

- ☐ Fruits (exception may be berries)

Depending on your current food intake, you may be able to eliminate all these foods at once in the first week of starting the MRP, or you will go on a gentle and progressive elimination, which allows your body to slowly adapt to the changes in available fuels; to slowly switch from burning carbohydrates as the main fuel to burning fat and producing ketones.

I recommend the following elimination schedule:

One Week Elimination (AKA Hard Core):

- ☐ Week 1: sugar, vegetable oils and all processed foods, milk, grains, starchy vegetables and legumes. Limit the amount of fruits and choose mostly organic berries.

Two Weeks Elimination:

- ☐ Week 1: sugar, vegetable oils and all processed foods, milk and grains.

- ☐ Week 2: starchy vegetables and legumes. Limit the amount of fruits and choose mostly organic berries.

Three Weeks Elimination:

☐ Week 1: sugar, vegetable oils and all processed foods.

☐ Week 2: milk and grains.

☐ Week 3: starchy vegetables and legumes. Limit the amount of fruits and choose mostly organic berries.

Your Whole Foods MRP Shopping List

Greens and non-starchy vegetables (carbohydrates):

☐ Artichoke

☐ Artichoke hearts

☐ Asparagus

☐ Bamboo shoots

☐ Beets*

☐ Broccoli

☐ Brussels sprouts

☐ Bell peppers

☐ Cabbage (green, bok choy, Chinese)

☐ Carrots*

☐ Cauliflower

☐ Celery

☐ Cucumber

☐ Daikon radish

☐ Eggplant

☐ Green Beans

☐ Greens (collard, kale, mustard, turnip)

☐ Hearts of palm

☐ Jicama

☐ Kohlrabi

☐ Leeks

☐ Mushrooms

☐ Okra

☐ Onions*

☐ Peppers

☐ Radishes

☐ Rutabaga

☐ Salad greens (chicory, endive, escarole, lettuce, romaine, spinach, arugula, radicchio, watercress)

☐ Squash (summer, spaghetti, zucchini)

☐ Sugar snap peas

☐ Swiss chard

☐ Tomato*

☐ Turnips*

☐ Water chestnut

*Some vegetables like carrots, beets, and onions, when cooked, release more of their sugar content, so go easy on those. Until you adapt to burning fat, you may omit them altogether.

Animal food (protein):

- [ ] Eggs from free range chickens
- [ ] Whole chicken
- [ ] Chicken thigh
- [ ] Chicken wings
- [ ] Chicken liver*
- [ ] Chicken gizzards*
- [ ] Chicken feet (for stock making)*
- [ ] Whole turkey and all its derivatives

- [ ] Sardines
- [ ] Herring
- [ ] Mackerel
- [ ] Trout
- [ ] Wild salmon
- [ ] Alaskan Sockeye
- [ ] Other wild caught fish
- [ ] Seafood
- [ ] Beef all cuts

- [ ] Beef organs (liver, tongue, kidney)*
- [ ] Beef bones for stock making*
- [ ] Pork, all cuts
- [ ] Pork organs (liver, kidney, heart)*, including bacon
- [ ] Lamb all cuts, including organs*
- [ ] Rabbit
- [ ] Sheep

* Particularly important to incorporate when following the gut reset protocol.

Animal and plant fats:

- [ ] Butter, preferably from grass-fed cows
- [ ] Ghee
- [ ] Lard
- [ ] Tallow

- [ ] Chicken, duck, goat, lamb fat (usually saved from roasting)
- [ ] Avocado
- [ ] Coconut oil/butter

- [ ] Cacao butter
- [ ] Olive oil
- [ ] Flax seed oil
- [ ] Hemp seed oil

Dairy products (preferably from grass fed cows):

- ☐ Cheese (look below for an extensive list)
- ☐ Yogurt
- ☐ Kefir
- ☐ Whey
- ☐ Sour cream
- ☐ Fresh heavy cream
- ☐ Butter and ghee

Cheese:

- ☐ Asiago cheese
- ☐ Brie
- ☐ Camembert
- ☐ Cheddar
- ☐ Cottage cheese
- ☐ Dubliner
- ☐ Emmental
- ☐ Feta
- ☐ Gorgonzola
- ☐ Gouda
- ☐ Gruyere
- ☐ Havarti
- ☐ Monterey Jack
- ☐ Labneh
- ☐ Mozzarella
- ☐ Mascarpone
- ☐ Parmesan
- ☐ Provolone
- ☐ Pecorino
- ☐ Queso blanco
- ☐ Roquefort
- ☐ Ricotta
- ☐ Stilton

Nuts and seeds:

- ☐ Almonds
- ☐ Brazil nuts*
- ☐ Cashews
- ☐ Coconuts*
- ☐ Macadamias*
- ☐ Pine nuts*
- ☐ Pistachios
- ☐ Pecans*
- ☐ Walnuts*
- ☐ Hazelnuts
- ☐ Sesame seeds*
- ☐ Sunflower seeds*
- ☐ Pumpkin seeds*
- ☐ Hemp seeds*
- ☐ Flax seeds*
- ☐ Chia seeds*

* Most MRP friendly, as they are lower in carbs, higher in fats and moderate in protein. In the resources section, you will find a side by side nut comparison table, listing their macronutrient breakdown.

Herbs and spices:

☐ Allspice

☐ Basil

☐ Cardamom

☐ Cumin

☐ Coriander

☐ Cinnamon

☐ Celery seed

☐ Dill

☐ Fenugreek

☐ Garlic

☐ Ginger

☐ Curry (red, green, yellow)

☐ Oregano

☐ Cilantro

☐ Nutmeg

☐ Rosemary

☐ Thyme

☐ Tarragon

☐ Garam masala

☐ Turmeric

☐ Cayenne pepper

☐ Peppercorns

☐ Bay leaf

☐ Hungarian paprika

☐ Chili powder

☐ Parsley

☐ Celtic sea salt

☐ Himalayan crystal salt

☐ Raw apple cider vinegar

☐ Lemon

☐ Limes

Please refer to the resources section for a table of selected nuts and cheeses with their caloric and macronutrient composition.

Now, what will you eat and how will figure out what goes on your plate?

Before you get into the fine tuning phase, when you start to keep track of the macros and measure blood sugar and blood ketones, use this simple rule:

☐ Choose 3 or more foods from the carbohydrates list (e.g. mixed greens, green onion, and radishes for a salad, asparagus as a side of cooked vegetables). In other words, fill up on as many vegetables as you like.

☐ Choose 1 (max 3) from the protein list (e.g. eggs and cheese). Eat enough protein so you feel satiated.

☐ Choose as much fat as you'd like (e.g. olive oil, olives and avocados, for the salad, coconut oil to cook the cheesy eggs, drizzle olive oil over the grilled asparagus). Same rule applies to fat, there is no limit, add as much as you need so the food you eat tastes good and you feel satisfied.

☐ Add any fresh herbs or dry spices to flavor the food.

The main goal of this phase, as well as the long term goal, is to make meals that you love. Although food is medicine, food is information, food has a hormonal effect on the body; food is also pleasure. You can't eat, not for the long run, food you don't love. That requires willpower and the "willpower tank" is small and empties fast. You will see, as you clean up your taste buds, add more fat, salt and spices, to your diet, you will begin to love the foods you didn't when you first started. You will eat less and feel satisfied. You will not feel deprived; it will all come effortlessly and naturally. Food will not stress you out anymore. It will not occupy all of your brain space, as it probably does now. I promise you. You will be at peace, not only with fat, but with food as well. You will live at a whole new dimension, at least with regards to food and energy!

During the adaptation phase, the easiest way to go about your meals and meal planning is to think of eating, by volume, more plant foods (non-starchy vegetables and green leafy vegetables) than anything else; while most of the energy (calories) of your meals will be supplied by fat. In other words, you eat liberal amounts of fat coming from olive oil, olives, avocado, coconut oil and butter. And that is aside from the fat that comes naturally with the animal protein you'll eat. With regards to protein or animal foods, you will consume them mostly according to your hunger. Chances are, at this stage, you will eat slightly more protein than you will in the long term, but do not worry about that now.

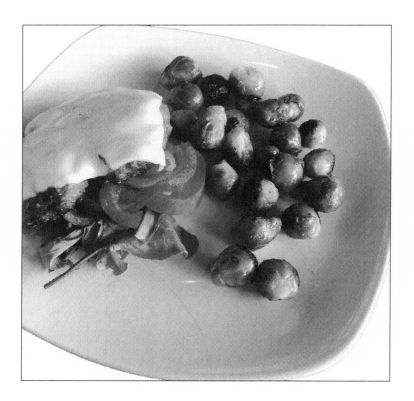

Should you snack?

During the adaptation period, and even for the first three or sometimes more months while embarking on low carbohydrate, high fat eating, you will still have difficulty regulating blood sugar and you may need to snack more often. However, overtime, your blood sugars, hunger and appetite will stabilize, and you will find yourself not having to snack as often, if at all.

When you need a snack, you can choose nuts or seeds (and their butters), cheese, avocado, berries, cucumbers, bell peppers, celery sticks with guacamole, heavy cream, fat-coffee or tea.

How about dining out?

Eating out, socializing and traveling can be stressful, especially at the beginning. You may find it difficult to order off the menu. You may have a hard time asking the kitchen to accommodate your dietary requests. You may find yourself being the "odd one."

As always, mindset is the first step in health transformation. You will need to work on your belief around this way of eating. Do not be afraid to ask for what you need. If you think it is odd then people around you will think it is odd. Be natural about it, as though this is the natural way to eat, because it is!

In the resources section of the book, I'm providing you with some tips that will make traveling and socializing not only easier, but eventually enjoyable, guilt free, stress free, and part of life you will be looking forward to.

After about 3 to 4 weeks, when this way of eating becomes more comfortable and it's somewhat easy for you to make your food selection, it's time to move to phase two: "fine tuning." Do not rush into this; take your time to adapt, both your mind as well as your body to eating this way, before going to the fine-tuning phase, as this is a little more stressful.

Phase 1: Initiation And Adaptation, At A Glance.

☐ Get the shopping list and familiarize yourself with the foods you'll be buying

☐ Eliminate insulinogenic carbs (sugar, grains, starches, legumes, milk and fruits)

☐ Eat protein and natural fats to satiety

☐ Eat only if hungry (try to avoid snacking if not absolutely hungry)

☐ Look at the one week menu and follow it as is, or adapted to your food likes and dislikes. Use it as startup guide

☐ Plan ahead; shop and cook for at least 3 days in advance

Phase 2: Fine tuning

During this phase, the goal is to become more precise about your macros, so you can fine tune the diet to help you reach your specific health goals. You want to determine your unique carbohydrate tolerance and protein threshold, and the remains of your energy needs will be met by fat.

The easiest way to do this is to track your food intake. Up to this point, you eliminated the insulinogenic carbs. Now, it's time for you to weigh the food and to log it into a nutrition app. This will allow you to see what your macros are at this time, 3 or more weeks into the MRP. Up to this point you allowed hunger and satiety to control your food intake. Intuitive eating! Please continue to follow your body's signals, do not eat if you are not hungry just to hit your macro targets. NO!

You first goal is to consume:

- < 50 g of NC per day.

- 0.6-1 g protein/pound lean body weight. You'll go for the higher range if you are more physically active and for the lower range if you are less active.

- Fat remains liberal, and guided by satiety.

Note: Too much protein will impair your ability to enter or stay in nutritional ketosis. Testing your blood sugar and ketones will help you determine your protein threshold as well as carbohydrate tolerance. For example, you may be eating 30 grams of NC a day, but you do not find yourself in NK (with ketone levels in the range of 0.5-5 mM), then you will need to look closer at the amount of protein you consume and dial it down. Chances are you are eating more than what your body needs, and the excess amino acids become a source of glucose and impair your fat burning ability.

How do you know you are ready for the fine tuning phase?

To begin this phase, you need to feel comfortable with this new way of eating. It must come naturally to put together your low carb, high fat meals. It no longer feels new, foreign or strange. You have sustained energy, and hunger is not running your life; in other words, if you don't need to eat right away when you feel hungry, you can ride the hunger wave and still have energy. Later, when you get to eat, you don't over eat. You are calm around food. You have good energy output in your workouts; you are even able to work out while fasting. Sleep is good, and you may actually notice that you require less sleep. You are less stiff and achy. Most importantly is the energy: you have a constant flow of energy. It's almost strange that you have energy and don't care to eat very much, in fact it comes naturally not to eat your breakfast or to skip your lunch and go straight to dinner, especially on busy days, when you are engaged in meaningful projects.

If this is not how you feel yet, do not start the fine tuning phase. You need to spend more time in the adaptation phase.

I spent 3 years on this phase. Yes, for the first three years of my healing with high fat low carb foods, I followed a gut healing protocol similar to GRP and never even cared to know the macro ratios. In fact, it is not a "must" to know your macros, as your body will take you intuitively into the macros that you thrive on. However, the fine tuning is important, too—especially when it comes to addressing metabolic syndrome, diabetes, cancer, and neurological disorders; when you have a very specific disease you are targeting with the MRP.

Food logging and macro tracking.

I recommend using the nutrient tracker Cronometer. I find it to be one of the best on the market for someone following a diet such as the MRP. It not only provides you with a nice macronutrient analyses, but it also gives all the minerals, vitamins, and fatty acids; it is very comprehensive. You will love it. When you create your account in Cronometer, you input your age, weight, height and activity level, as well as your goal (to maintain, gain or lose weight). It will provide your calculated Resting Energy Expenditure (they use the Mifflin equation, one of the most accurate out there), as well as the total calories to consume to meet your weight goal you've set at the beginning.

It also allows you to pick the dietary plan you'd like to follow (e.g. keto strict, relaxed, moderate). I am happy to let you know that the founder of the company and I developed a nice relationship over time and he provided me with a customized version of the app, to better support you in your efforts to fine tune the MRP. To create a free account you can go to www.cronometer.com/telecan.

You may ask why I'm talking about calories when I say that what matters is the macronutrient ratio, and how they interact with the hormones that regulate metabolism when it comes to metabolic health and weigh management. The short answer is to calculate macro ratios.

There are two distinct ways we can look at macronutrients: one is absolute value, and the other one is percentages based on caloric value. They are both correct. One looks at grams of macros. The other one looks at percent of calories from macros in reference to total energy intake.

	Absolute value grams	Caloric value calories	Percent %
Net carbs	30	120	7%
Protein	60	240	15%
Fat	130	1170	77%
Total daily intake		1530	100%

If you find yourself constantly on a positive energy balance while keeping carbs low and protein moderate, you may stop losing weight or body fat, as you will burn more of the dietary fat than your own body fat.

In my clinical experience, most women that were chronic dieters see the most results at around 30 g NC per day with 50-60 g of protein per day and around 100-130 g of fat. That translates into about 1200-1500 caloric intake per day, which allows them to lose about 0.5 lbs./week, and have good glycemic control while in nutritional ketosis for the greater part of the day.

The way to do it is to "lock in" the first two macronutrients (carbs and protein), and the third one (fat) goes as high as necessary to meet energy demands. Some days you'll need more energy, some days less; so, your calories will go up and down with the fat.

Depending on your age, activity level, insulin sensitivity, hormonal balance and gender, you may be able to eat more than 50 g of NC/day and still be in the nu-tritional ketosis zone, or you may need to keep it as low as 20 g NC/day. Each person responds differently. One thing is certain: the longer you stay on less than 50 g NC/day, the more metabolically flexible you become and your body will switch easily from burning carbs to burning fat. Then you'll no longer feel big energy fluctuations or extreme hunger.

So, in order to determine your unique carb and protein tolerance, it's import-ant that you begin to weigh your food, log it, and start testing your blood sugar and ketones.

Full disclosure: This phase is time consuming and tiring. With time and practice, it becomes easier. Once you learn your body's response to carbs and proteins, you learn to eyeball your portions; you will not need to weigh, measure food, document and test all of the time. You may do it only occasionally.

Personally, I don't like this phase. I don't stay on it for more than a few weeks to a month at a time, and that's only when I train for a long bike ride or I have other major life changes that require fine tuning.

Unless managing type I or type II diabetes, or cancer and neurological disease are one of your goals, you will not need to spend too much time on this phase either.

Nevertheless, you will need to fine tune at least once per year.

When you fine tune for the first time, give yourself 1-3 months to do it.

Do not let this phase overpower your body's signals or to take the joy of eating out of your life.

Blood Sugar and Ketone Testing.

I recommend using a meter that allows you to test both. You will use different strips: one for glucose and one for ketones (beta hydroxybutyrate).

You will want to test your fasting levels, as well as your levels after meals (post-prandial) at various intervals between meals. Keep a log of the readings. In fact, you can add the ketone and glucose readings to the biomarkers section in Cronometer.

There are few meters on the market that are good. The one I personally use and I recommend to my clients is Nova Max Plus. The other one I'm aware of is Precision Xtra made by Abbott. You can purchase either directly from the man-ufacturer or from Amazon. The blood glucose strips are inexpensive, $ 0.10 - 0.15 per strip, but the ketone ones are pricier, $1.50 - 1.70 per strip. If you are diabetic or pre-diabetic, you may be able to get them covered by your medical insurance. If that is the case, ask your doctor for a prescription. To give you an idea of the cost, when I test my glucose and ketones for a month, I spend between $80-$90 for 100 blood sugar strips and 40 ketone strips combined.

I recommend working with a qualified coach or practitioner that is well versed in nutritional ketosis that will be able to guide you through this process.

Below you have a visual representation of blood or ketone testing.

> TIP: Pre-plan your meals the night before. First, create your menu for the day in Cronometer so it meets your macro targets. Then, weigh the food and have it ready to serve the next day, or weigh it right before you eat. Before and after you eat, test your blood sugar and blood ketones to eval-uate your body's response to the meal. Rather than eating, logging and then finding out afterwards that you were way above your targets, this way allows you to fine tune your macros more rapidly and effectively. It's the proactive not the reactive way. This will shorten the fine tuning phase.

How to test BS and BK: a step by step guide

1. Wash your hands

2. Insert the needle in the lancet device and adjust for how deep it needs to prick (thick skin = higher number)

3. Insert the testing strip in the meter

4. Prick your finger. Choose the side of the finger, as it is less painful

5. Press around the prick to express a good drop of blood. If you have poor circulation, warm up your fingers before testing; it helps bring more blood to the fingers

6. Touch the blood droplet to the edge of the strip. Make sure the blood runs through the small canal on the strip all the way to the end and that it makes a beep (if the sound feature is on). For ketone readings, you will need a bit more blood than for the glucose

7. In 5 and 10 seconds you will have the results for the blood sugar and the blood ketones, respectively

8. Keep a log with the time, the value and if it was fasting or post-prandial

Add Intermittent Fasting.

This step is optional; however it is very powerful.

In fact, when you follow the MRP for a while, even before you start the fine tuning phase, you will find yourself less hungry, and you will naturally incorporate various forms of fasting without even noticing, simply by default. It's a natural progression of things.

> The default of the carb burner is over eating,
> and that of the fat burner is fasting.

Let me illustrate this, as you already know I love analogies. You are listening to music, and with time, you realize how much you like this particular rock band; all you want to listen to is their music. So, you begin searching and find a radio station that plays only this rock band's music. Now, you are super happy; you found the best radio station and you can listen to their music as much as you like. But you want more. So what do you do? You search to see if they perform live concerts. Of course they do, so you go to see them live in concert. That is the fullest experience you could possibly dream of having.

Fasting is the equivalent of going to the live concert of your favorite rock band. It is the natural progression of everything that happened before. Listening to music is the equivalent of reading this book, listening to podcasts, learning about food and its role in healing. As you become more aware of the food-health-body connection, you begin to choose your food more carefully, eat fresh whole foods, free of sugar, additives, and vegetable oils, organic, and non-GMO. This is like discovering your favorite rock band. Eating high fat, low carb foods is like finding the radio station that plays only your favorite rock band's music. Now, going to see them live in concert is the next logical step. Fasting is just like going to the live concert.

The easiest fast protocol to incorporate into anyone's lifestyle is the intermittent fasting (IF) in the form of a compressed eating window.

How to get started with IF:

1. Begin to track when you eat

   - first meal of the day,

   - last meal of the day,

   - when and how often you snack.

2. Decide whether you want to compress the eating time from breakfast up or from dinner down, or if you need to work on both ends. In other words, you may begin by eating your breakfast every day half an hour later than your usual time, until you eat your first meal of the day somewhere between 12 and 1pm. Or, if you choose to eat an early breakfast and end 8 hours later, you will begin to move your dinner down by 30-60 min each night until you reach your desired time.

3. Determine the time you'll have your last meal, so it won't be later than 6 to 8 hours from your first meal. In our example, if you have your first meal at 12pm, you will have your dinner no later than 8 PM. Preferably, give yourself about three hours between the last meal of the day and the time you go to bed.

What will you consume during the fasting state (before noon or after 3 pm)?

One way to stay in a fasted state is to consume only water and unsweetened tea. Another option is to do a fat fast. You may add to your hot coffee or tea fats, such as butter, coconut oil, or MCT oil and blend them together. A classic example of this is Dave Asprey's bulletproof coffee. I'm providing a recipe for a fat coffee in the recipes section.

For longer fasts (24 hour or longer), I recommend water, fat, meat/bone stock and fermented beverages (kvass, sauerkraut juice).

Other ways of intermittent fasting can be a 24-hour fast—dinner to dinner, for example. You can do it two or three times in a week.

As you become more fat adapted, occasionally you may incorporate 3 to 5 days of water-fat-broth fasting. I strongly recommend when you do this to do it with your medical doctor's approval and close supervision, especially if you are taking multiple medications to manage chronic diseases, and if you are taking insulin and other hypoglycemic agents for blood sugar control.

Keep in mind, longer fasts and more frequent fasts have a therapeutic effect. They allow the body to self-clean and they support deep cellular detox and healing. Over time, fasting will become easier, as your overall hunger will diminish; you'll be satisfied with less food, while your body will get its energy needs from your stored fat. Since you will be eating less food, choosing the most nutrient dense foods is key to successfully incorporating fasting and low carbs into your diet.

Phase 2: Fine Tuning, At A Glance.

☐ Track your food intake

☐ Determine your macros. Use the following guidelines to get started:

- NC (net carbohydrates) <50 g/day

- Protein: 0.6 -1 g/pound of lean body weight

- Fat eat to satiety

☐ Test blood glucose

☐ Test blood ketones

☐ Incorporate intermittent fasting

Phase 3: Maintenance.

This phase, as the name implies, is to be followed for the rest of your life, or for as long as you see that this way of eating is benefiting you. This is a lifestyle not a diet; you will have to adapt it to the changes your body will go through as you grow older, or as you become more active.

Occasionally, you will reevaluate and determine if your macros need adjustments. You'll periodically measure laboratory biomarkers; your body composition; try on your "before outfit;" and, hopefully, 6 months, one year or more into it, you'll see many changes in your health, looks and energy.

An important element in the maintenance phase is something I like to refer to as Feast - Famine Ancestral Cycles (FFAC).

Our ancestors went from periods of fasting to periods of feasting. I believe that served an important role in our evolution and metabolic function; hence, there is value in it and we can adapt it to our lifestyle today.

One thing that was different about ancestral eating was the unpredictability of meal timing. There was no set or expected time for eating; it was more of a sporadic and random event. I believe this is a key factor in human health, resilience and even the ability to lose or maintain weight. I believe too much stability and comfort (I mean biological comfort) may not be all that good for us. This is pure speculation, my personal conclusion based on all my readings, learnings and doings, not based on any scientific studies. I just feel that when we have too much comfort, for some reason, it is not good for our health. If we are never hungry (regular meals), never cold, never hot (climate controlled environment), never dirty (anti-microbial soaps), never suntanned (sun screen protectors) etc. our biology gets "stunted." It's like we don't allow this amazing biological machine, the human body, to function at its full potential.

The point I'm trying to make is that there is a benefit in taking our body out of its comfort zone. Practicing unpredictable eating may be the key to optimizing our metabolism, increasing our resilience, and keeping a healthy body and mind. Your body perhaps shouldn't get too comfortable with the time you always eat, what you eat and how much you eat.

This is a very similar approach to the one used for exercise. You periodically have to change your routines so your body doesn't adapt to it. That's, of course, if you want to maximize the results from your gym workout.

How can you mimic the FFAC?

Think that for a very long time in your life you found yourself in a feast-like state. For years and years you ate 3 regular meals a day and perhaps 2-3 snacks. Over time, you accumulated considerable fat reserves and your health may be deteriorating.

Now, you are going to follow the metabolic reset protocol, which mimics fasting times. After following the low-carb, high-fat diet for six months to a year, you may begin to see significant metabolic reset. Now, may be a good time to add periods of feasting. During those you eat more food as well as more carbohydrates. Those feasting times can be of shorter or longer duration. You may take certain social events, like a birthday or wedding or an office party, and decide that those are your feast times.

Even during such events, it's important to keep in mind that the quality of food is very important. Do not allow "food-like substances" back onto your plate or into your body!

On a feast day, you can go up with your carbs to two or even three times more than on your regular days. I can't stress it enough how important it is to make those carbs whole foods carbs; it may be sweet potatoes, winter squashes, quinoa, lentils, or fruits.

After a feast day, you can throw in a 24-hour fast. Or before a feast day, imagine that you are the hunter or gatherer that has no food left, and you are out there looking to hunt or to gather food. This is a situation that we can imagine our ancestors were in often. So, you may be more physically active outdoors while fasting and the next day (after you have caught your next meal), you are going to feast on it. The pre-feast can be a 24- or 72-hour fast, with or without more intense activity. That's pushing your body to its limits, while creating resilience and a need to survive. This approach (fasted exercise) may work better for athletic men and women.

Depending on your weight and health, you will adapt the FFAC to make it work for you. However, you will most likely not need to incorporate FFAC for the first 6-12 months of starting the MRP.

Dr. Dan Pompa has developed a protocol which aims to add variability to the diet: it's called 5:1:1 schedule. He suggests 5 days a week you eat your usual low carb, high fat menu. 1 day a week you do a complete fast. Another 1 day a week you do a feast.

I believe that adding various forms of intermittent fasting to the low carb-high fat plan and random feasting days can be the key to long term success.

Personally, I follow local and seasonal eating. In Florida, where I live, I eat a bit more fruits in the summer, as they are more abundant, and less over the winter. I do daily IF with a compressed eating window of 4-8 hours. Occasionally, I throw in a 24-hour fast (dinner to dinner) and I sprinkle some feast days very randomly, not preplanned. This works for me.

With my private clients, I help them develop their unique FFAC.

The more insulin resistant you are or the more weight you need to lose, the longer you'll need to wait to add random feasting days to your regimen.

Phase 3: Maintenance, At A Glance.

☐ *Maintain a low carb, moderate protein, high fat diet long term to help you reach your goals (weight, health, energy, performance)*

☐ *Periodically check biomarkers (blood sugar, blood ketones, body composition as well as pertinent laboratory tests)*

☐ *Practice intermittent fasting*

☐ *Randomly add FFAC*

Must Know About the MRP:

Eat more salt.

When following a diet low in insulinogenic carbohydrates, you have higher requirements for sodium.[21] Insulin has a sodium retention effect. When insulin levels remain low (as a result of carb restriction or fasting), the body loses more sodium via urine (natriuresis); hence, the need to increase sodium consumption. If you don't, your blood volume drops and that affects blood pressure which can lead to orthostatic hypotension (sudden drop in blood pressure, when standing up), dizziness, fainting or fatigue.

Many of the so called "keto flu" symptoms are due to low sodium and an imbalance in the other electrolytes (potassium, magnesium, calcium). When salt is not added back into the diet, the kidneys compensate for that and begin to waste potassium as a compensatory mechanism. Low potassium levels affect heart and skeletal muscle contractions (irregular heartbeats, muscle cramps).

To prevent all of these, you must add more salt to your diet. *I know first I'm telling you to Make Peace with FAT & EAT MORE FAT and now I'm telling you to Make Peace with SALT & EAT MORE SALT! Looks like you've got to unlearn everything you've been taught all these years!*

Ways to add more salt to your diet:

☐ add salt to your foods; make sure it tastes salty

☐ drink and eat fermented beverages/foods

☐ have the classic homemade meat/bone stock (this will not only be high in sodium, but it also has potassium and other minerals leaching from the bones and meat).

How much salt should you add?

☐ Start with by adding 1-2 g of sodium per day. Pay attention to how you feel. If your ankles get swollen, cut back. Note: ¼ tsp. Himalayan salt has 420 mg of Na.

☐ If you exercise or work in the yard and sweat profusely, have salt 30 min before the exercise; drink bone broth or a fermented juice like sauerkraut juice.

☐ If the addition of sodium and potassium are not enough to prevent muscle spasms and cramps, you may consider adding magnesium supplements as well.

Rapid and transient increase in uric acid.

You may see a rapid increase in blood uric acid in the first few weeks of initiating carb restriction. That is due to changes in the way the kidneys work. Basically, during the adaptation phase, kidneys filter out ketones and hold off uric acid. After about 4-6 weeks, blood uric acid comes back to normal. This is a normal part of the adaptation to nutritional ketosis, and it is safe for most people. [21] However, if you have gout or a propensity towards it, you may want to keep this in mind, as it can trigger an attack and you may need medical intervention. It is best in this case to avoid going on and off the low carb plan.

A transient increase in cholesterol (total and LDL).

During major weight loss (30 pounds or more), we can see a transient increase in total cholesterol. As Dr. Voleck explains in his book, *"THE ART AND SCIENCE OF LOW CARBOHYDRATE LIVING,"* a small amount of cholesterol is stored inside the adipose tissue. As a person loses a significant amount of weight (around 30 pounds), some of the cholesterol trapped inside the adipose tissue is released in the blood stream and it appears to be taken to the liver for clearance in the LDL particles; hence, the transient rise in both total cholesterol and LDL is noted. Once the fat loss stops, the cholesterol and LDL go back to what now becomes the post weight-loss normal cholesterol for that person. So, if you are doing a lipid test during this time, do not panic if the numbers appear to be higher. It's part of the fat loss process. Retest again once you reach weight maintenance, or about three months into the diet.

NOTE: Although your total cholesterol and LDL may be high during this major weight loss phase, your triglycerides are probably very low (in the 60-70s) and your HbA1C may have dropped significantly; that is an indicator that your body responds to the MRP. If cardiovascular disease is your concern, please check with a cardiologist and test particle size cholesterol as well as other known cardiovascular risk factors.

A simple formula I am using to assess cholesterol and its atherogenic effect, if a particle size report is not available is:

☐ Divide HDL by Total Cholesterol X 100. A good result is >24%

☐ Divide total triglycerides by HDL. A good result is <2

Gallbladder stones genesis.

If not enough fat is consumed, while starting to eat low carb, and significant weight loss takes place, the person may develop gallbladder stones.

The liver makes bile salts using cholesterol. Bile salts are a major component of the bile, which is stored inside the gallbladder. When a fatty meal is consumed, bile is excreted into the small intestine and is used for fat emulsification and assists with fat digestion. Part of the bile and cholesterol will leave the body via stools, and part gets recycled back to the liver. Consumption of dietary fat is what triggers the gallbladder to contract and release the bile.

Here's the catch: if the cholesterol is stored inside the gallbladder as bile salts, but you are not eating enough fat to stimulate the bladder to empty regularly, those bile salts remain in the gallbladder and can turn into stones; hence, you are at risk of forming gallbladder stones. To prevent this from happening, all you need to do is to eat more fat.

That's one more reason for you to make peace with fat and eat more of it.

To prevent gallbladder stone formation, it is recommended to consume a minimum of 30 g of fat a day, which assures the gallbladder is stimulated and releases the bile with its cholesterol-rich salts. That shouldn't be too difficult to get, as a meal on the MRP supplies that much fat or more.

Exercise and the MRP.

Do not change your exercise routine when you start the MRP. Continue with whatever exercise plan you had, as if nothing has changed in your diet. Changing both exercise and diet at the same time is the recipe for failure.

If you are not exercising, wait until you are well adapted to burning fat and then add exercise. Just by following the MRP, most likely, you'll lose some weight, you'll have less pain and more energy; so, adding planned exercise later will make more sense.

In the beginning stages of the MRP, be mindful of moving your body naturally and habitually. More about movement and exercise will come in the next chapter: "Healing Beyond Food."

As you can see, there are many intricacies and little details one needs to pay attention to when starting the MRP or any low carb diet that induces ketogenesis.

Glycemic Index (GI) and Glycemic Load (GL).

You may come across books, blogs, practitioners, etc. that will bring up GI and GL when they talk about dietary interventions to address metabolic disorders, such as those we've been discussing in this book.

I think that the GI and GL are confusing and often misleading. Here's an example of a misleading use of GI/GL: peanut M&M's have a GI of 33 and a GL of 6, which makes them good, as a GL less than 10 and GI less than 55 are considered to be low. In fact, according to this, M&M's are better than bananas as a banana (120 g serving) has a GI of 51 and a GL of 11. I think you will agree with me that M&M's are food-like substances loaded with sugar and artificial colors. If I was to recommend for you to eat something that's high in insulinogenic carbs, I would for sure recommend a banana over M&M's. Hence, looking at a food based on its GI or GL is, in my opinion, misleading and it can get complicated.

I believe GI and GL have very little relevance to you, should you choose to follow the metabolic reset protocol; however, I also believe in making informed decisions. Hence, I will take time to explain the two concepts, and in the end you may decide if you are going to use them or not. Let's see what GI and GL are:

Glycemic index (GI) and glycemic load (GL) assess how a carbohydrate containing food influences blood glucose levels.

GI is a numerical system measuring how much of a rise in circulating blood sugar a carbohydrate triggers–the higher the number, the greater the blood sugar response. See the table below for GI and GL classification. The GI value tells you only how rapidly a particular carbohydrate turns into sugar and gets into your bloodstream. It doesn't tell you how much of that carbohydrate is in a serving of a particular food, which also affects the rise in blood sugar.

This disadvantage of the GI is addressed by using the GL.

The GL gives a numerical value indicating how a single serving of food affects blood sugar. It multiplies the amount of carbohydrates found in a serving of food with that food's GI and divides that number by 100. [40]

	High	Medium	Low
Glycemic Index (GI)	>70	59-69	<55
Glycemic Load (GL)	>20	11-19	<10

For example, watermelon has a high GI of 72 and a low GL of 4. Looking at the GI, watermelon fits in the high classification. If we go by the GL, watermelon is "safe" to eat, as the GL is low. Conflicting right? Here's why: the GL is calculated using the amount of carbs in a single serving of watermelon, or 120 g. To help put that into perspective, that's less than a cup of diced watermelon; a full cup weighs 150 g. The serving size, on which the GL is based, is very small. Chances are that most people consume more than 120 g of watermelon at a time; especially knowing that it is a low GL food, when in fact it spikes both sugar and insulin significantly.

Can you see how using GL can be misleading? It gives a false sense of security. When we keep in mind that the insulin resistant person is "carbohydrate intolerant," it is only logical that we need to remove all carbs that trigger an insulin spike (aka. insulinogenic carbs), independent of their assigned GI or GL values.

The main objective of the MRP is to reduce the overall need for insulin secretion. The fastest way to achieve that is through elimination of insulinogenic carbs and through fasting. This is not to say that maintaining normal blood sugar is irrelevant. No.

It is important that we maintain normal blood sugar levels, as chronically elevated blood glucose affects, in a negative way, every cell in the body, from nerves to tiny blood vessels in your kidney, eyes, and cardiovascular system.

The beauty of following the MRP is that it helps keep blood sugar and blood insulin levels low, by following one simple elimination criteria. I find it much simpler to eliminate all insulinogenic carbohydrates and to only keep track of one value: Net Carbs. The carbs that are part of the MRP (greens, non-starchy vegetables, nuts, seeds and cheese) are all low GI and GL, so no need to even look at their value.

That is why I don't use or recommend the GI or the GL; however, if it is something you like to use, feel free to do it, as this is your journey. I thought I would share with you my thoughts on it, as many practitioners out there are still using it, and you may have heard about it and probably wonder if it's something worth learning and using.

This concludes the MRP section. Next I'll be talking about the gut reset protocol (GRP).

PART 5.2:
THE GUT RESET PROTOCOL (GRP)

The GRP includes two levels of intervention: one aims to support optimal enterocyte function (a cellular approach) and the other one focuses on rebalancing the gut flora (the main controller of gut health and overall health).

Restoring the enterocyte function and gut integrity is a three-fold approach: re-move, re-build and re-inoculate.

#1. Re-Move: during this phase, you will eliminate all foods containing di - and polysaccharides, aside from processed foods, which you've already started to eliminate during the pantry and refrigerator cleaning phase.

☐ all processed foods (including vegetable oils and margarines)

☐ sugar

☐ grains

☐ legumes

☐ starches

☐ milk

#2. Re-Build: during this phase, you will focus on nourishing your gut and, by extent, your body. You'll do this by adding foods that provide easily absorbable amino acids and fats.

☐ joints, bones and bone marrow, fat, and organ meats.

#3. Re-Inoculate: the focus here is on re-inoculation and re-balancing of the gut flora. This is mainly done by:

☐ the addition of fermented foods (lacto-fermented vegetables, fermented dairy products and even meats)

☐ therapeutic strength probiotics

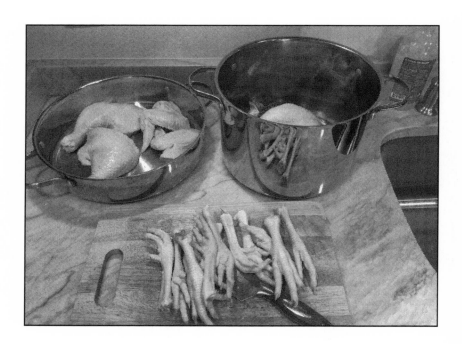

This is your very simple GRP shopping list:

- ☐ Fresh leafy greens and non-starchy vegetables

- ☐ Fresh eggs (from pasture raised chickens)

- ☐ Fresh or frozen meats and fish (not smoked or canned)

- ☐ Shellfish

- ☐ Cheese, preferably from grass fed cows

- ☐ Raw nuts and seeds

- ☐ Organic cream, butter and ghee, preferably from grass fed cows

- ☐ Lard, beef tallow, and other animal fats rendered from cooking

- ☐ Olive oil, coconut oil, cacao butter

- ☐ Avocado

- ☐ Garlic, Celtic Sea Salt or Himalayan Crystal Salt

- ☐ Spices and herbs

- ☐ Berries and other fruits you find in your local area (fully ripened)

- ☐ Honey

Comprehensive GRP shopping list

Greens and non-starchy vegetables (carbohydrates):

- ☐ Artichoke
- ☐ Artichoke hearts
- ☐ Asparagus
- ☐ Bamboo shoots
- ☐ Beets
- ☐ Broccoli
- ☐ Brussels sprouts
- ☐ Bell peppers
- ☐ Cabbage (green, bok choy, Chinese)
- ☐ Carrots
- ☐ Cauliflower
- ☐ Celery

- ☐ Cucumber
- ☐ Daikon radish
- ☐ Eggplant
- ☐ Green Beans
- ☐ Greens (collard, kale, mustard, turnip)
- ☐ Hearts of palm
- ☐ Jicama
- ☐ Kohlrabi
- ☐ Leeks
- ☐ Mushrooms
- ☐ Okra
- ☐ Onions

- ☐ Peppers
- ☐ Radishes
- ☐ Rutabaga
- ☐ Salad greens (chicory, endive, escarole, lettuce, romaine, spinach, arugula, radicchio, watercress)
- ☐ Squash (summer, spaghetti, zucchini)
- ☐ Sugar snap peas
- ☐ Swiss chard
- ☐ Tomato
- ☐ Turnips
- ☐ Water chestnut

Sweeteners:

- ☐ Honey
- ☐ Fresh or dry fruits

Animal foods (protein):

- ☐ Eggs from free range chickens
- ☐ Whole chicken
- ☐ Chicken thigh
- ☐ Chicken wings
- ☐ Chicken liver
- ☐ Chicken gizzards
- ☐ Chicken feet (for stock making)
- ☐ Whole turkey and all its derivatives
- ☐ Sardines
- ☐ Herring
- ☐ Mackerel
- ☐ Trout
- ☐ Wild salmon
- ☐ Alaskan Sockeye
- ☐ Other wild caught fish
- ☐ Seafood
- ☐ Beef all cuts
- ☐ Beef organs (liver, tongue, kidney)
- ☐ Beef bones (for stock making)
- ☐ Pork, all cuts, including bacon
- ☐ Pork organs (liver, kidney, heart)
- ☐ Lamb all cuts, including organs
- ☐ Rabbit
- ☐ Sheep

Animal and plant fat:

- ☐ Butter, preferably from grass fed cows
- ☐ Ghee
- ☐ Lard
- ☐ Tallow
- ☐ Chicken, duck, goat or lamb fat (usually saved from roasting)
- ☐ Avocado
- ☐ Coconut oil/butter
- ☐ Cacao butter
- ☐ Olive oil
- ☐ Flax seed oil
- ☐ Hemp seed oil

Dairy products (preferably from grass fed cows):

- ☐ Yogurt
- ☐ Kefir
- ☐ Whey
- ☐ Sour cream
- ☐ Fresh, heavy cream
- ☐ Butter
- ☐ Ghee

Cheese:

- ☐ Asiago cheese
- ☐ Brie
- ☐ Camembert
- ☐ Cheddar
- ☐ Cottage cheese
- ☐ Dubliner
- ☐ Emmental
- ☐ Feta

- ☐ Gorgonzola
- ☐ Gouda
- ☐ Gruyere
- ☐ Havarti
- ☐ Monterey Jack
- ☐ Labneh
- ☐ Mozzarella
- ☐ Mascarpone

- ☐ Parmesan
- ☐ Provolone
- ☐ Pecorino
- ☐ Queso blanco
- ☐ Roquefort
- ☐ Ricotta
- ☐ Stilton

Nuts and seeds:

- ☐ Almonds
- ☐ Brazil nuts
- ☐ Cashews
- ☐ Coconuts
- ☐ Macadamias
- ☐ Pine nuts

- ☐ Pistachios
- ☐ Pecans
- ☐ Walnuts
- ☐ Hazelnuts
- ☐ Sesame seeds
- ☐ Sunflower seeds

- ☐ Pumpkin seeds
- ☐ Hemp seeds
- ☐ Flax seeds
- ☐ Chia seeds

Fruits (carbohydrates):

- ☐ Apples
- ☐ Apricots
- ☐ Bananas
- ☐ Blueberries

- ☐ Blackberries
- ☐ Currant
- ☐ Cherise
- ☐ Cranberries

- ☐ Dates
- ☐ Durian
- ☐ Elderberry
- ☐ Fig

- [ ] Goji berry
- [ ] Grape/raisins
- [ ] Grapefruit
- [ ] Kiwi
- [ ] Lemon
- [ ] Lime
- [ ] Lychee
- [ ] Mango
- [ ] Melon (watermelon, cantaloupe, honeydew)
- [ ] Mulberry
- [ ] Nectarine
- [ ] Olive
- [ ] Orange
- [ ] Papaya
- [ ] Peach
- [ ] Pear
- [ ] Persimmon
- [ ] Plum/prune
- [ ] Pineapple
- [ ] Pomegranate
- [ ] Pomelo
- [ ] Raspberry
- [ ] Star fruit
- [ ] Strawberry
- [ ] Tamarind

Herbs and spices:

- [ ] Allspice
- [ ] Basil
- [ ] Cardamom
- [ ] Cumin
- [ ] Coriander
- [ ] Cinnamon
- [ ] Celery seed
- [ ] Dill
- [ ] Fenugreek
- [ ] Garlic
- [ ] Ginger
- [ ] Curry (red, green, yellow)
- [ ] Oregano
- [ ] Cilantro
- [ ] Nutmeg
- [ ] Rosemary
- [ ] Thyme
- [ ] Tarragon
- [ ] Garam masala
- [ ] Turmeric
- [ ] Cayenne pepper
- [ ] Peppercorns
- [ ] Bay leaf
- [ ] Hungarian paprika
- [ ] Chili powder
- [ ] Parsley
- [ ] Celtic sea salt
- [ ] Himalayan crystal salt
- [ ] Raw apple cider vinegar
- [ ] Lemon
- [ ] Limes

The best way to implement the GRP is to take the three phases all at the same time. As you begin to eliminate what's no longer serving you, you also begin to add what does and what supports healing of the gut flora. Don't see them as separate phases in time; they should be stuck on top of each other and morph into each other. In fact a better word to describe it is intertwined.

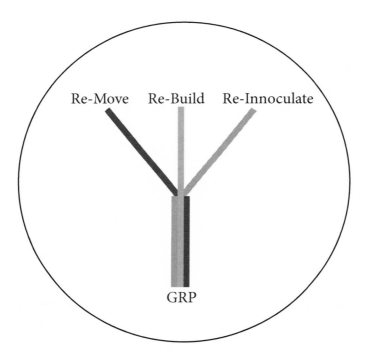

Next I will go over the step-by-step implementation process.

Phase 1: Re-Move:

☐ Focus on the elimination of "specific" carbohydrates. Refer to the shopping list to see what foods will become your source of carbohydrates.

☐ You may also eliminate raw vegetables and fruit, as their fiber may not be suited to your digestive tract.

☐ You may choose to eat all your plant foods in a cooked, moist state. This is similar to a low residue diet (low fiber diet).

This helps in two ways:

1. cooked plant foods are less irritating for the inflamed gut lining;

2. they are also more nourishing, so you may absorb more nutrients from them as opposed to the raw ones.

How long will you take to eliminate all the sugar, starches and grains from your diet?

It depends on you. It may go from 1 to 3 weeks. You set the tone to how fast you want to eliminate the "offenders." The faster you do it, the faster you'll begin to feel better; but, at the same time, the more difficult the transition. Some people take 1 week per food group, while others eliminate them all at once.

As long as you set a goal and you do it, you are heading in the right direction.

Below, you'll see three elimination plan schedules.

One Week Elimination:

☐ Week 1: sugar, vegetable oils and all processed foods, milk, grains, starchy vegetables and legumes

Two Weeks Elimination

☐ Week 1: sugar, vegetable oils and all processed foods, milk and grains

☐ Week 2: starchy vegetables and legumes

Three Weeks Elimination

☐ Week 1: sugar, vegetable oils and all processed foods

☐ Week 2: milk and grains

☐ Week 3: starchy vegetables and legumes

Pick the schedule that best fits your life and current situation. Some people can jump into it, while other like to dip their toes in first and then dive in. There is no right or wrong. Pick one plan, commit to it, set the intention, make it a "must," and go do it.

Phase 2: Re-Build:

☐ Add the nourishing animal foods (organ meats, bones, meat with its fat). This step is key to healing the gut lining.

☐ Make a chicken Stock/Broth. Begin by adding this from day 1. You will find the recipe in the resource section of the book. Keep in mind: you don't need to wait to eliminate all the foods described in phase 1 before you begin to add the gut nourishing and healing foods. These phases of the GRP overlap. While you may take 1 to 3 weeks and sometimes more to fully implement phase one, you will add the foods of phase 2 and 3 right from the beginning.

☐ Refer to the one week "done for you" whole foods menu, as it is a good representation of what you can eat on the GRP. Follow it as is, or adapt it to your food likes, dislikes and tolerances. Use it as blueprint to create your own GRP menu.

Phase 3: Re-Inoculate:

☐ Add fermented foods, such as the classic sauerkraut and its juice, lacto-fermented vegetables (like cucumbers or green tomatoes), fermented dairies (yogurt, kefir, if you don't have a known dairy allergy), and kvass.

o You can make your own or purchase them. If you choose to buy them, make sure they don't contain vinegar and are not pasteurized.

☐ Look in the recipes section for ferments recipes.

☐ It may be beneficial to start taking therapeutic strength probiotics, as well as soil microorganisms.

If you have not been eating fermented foods and/or taking therapeutic strength probiotics, I recommend you start adding the fermented foods gradually. Begin with small amounts and increase it progressively.

The addition of the "good" microbes has a "killing" effect on the pathogenic ones, which leads to the release of more toxins in the gut. These will absorb into your system and cause more ill effects at first. This phenomenon is known as the "die off reaction."

You can control this effect by introducing the ferments slowly, and gradually increasing the amount consumed, as tolerated.

I highly recommend working closely with a practitioner that will know how to guide you through this process.

Tips for GRP.

1. Keep a food-symptom log. It's very important to track what you eat and how you feel. For a sample food-symptoms log visit http://bit.ly/GRPFoodLog.

2. Start the day with water at room temperature; add apple cider vinegar to it or lemon juice, and a pinch of salt. Drink this or just plain water at room temperature for the first part of the morning, and don't eat right away; wait until you become hungry.

3. Eat as often as you need. Follow your hunger cues. Get in tune with your body. Eat only when you are truly hungry and stop when you are full. Pay attention to see if you eat out of boredom, anxiety, or for any other reason.

4. Make sure you have plenty of fat in your diet, as it is crucial for healing.

5. Consume daily meat/bone (chicken) stock. You can drink it as is, or add vegetables to it and serve it as a rich vegetable soup.

6. Add daily ferments to your meals.

7. Chew your food very well: 25-50 chews per mouthful. It will help you taste the food better, prepare it for digestion, improve digestion, and reduce gastric reflux. I keep reminding my 6 year old to chew well, as his stomach doesn't have teeth. I think most adults need the same reminder.

8. Avoid drinking and eating at the same time. It is best if you stop drinking 15 - 20 min before you eat and wait 1.5 - 2 hours to drink after a meal. If you need to drink sooner, that it's an indicator that the food was too salty, spicy or dry. When you eat moist foods, your need for water is slightly reduced.

9. Avoid using a microwave. Use traditional ways of cooking, like simmering, slow cooking, baking, sautéing, steaming, braising and, occasionally, grilling.

10. Incorporate daily gratitude, outdoor activities, sun and earth time. Emotions play a huge role in healing. Master your mind.

A Word About Food Quality.

GRP emphasizes the quality of the food more than the quantity. Make it a priority to connect with local farmers. Visit farmer's markets in your area. If you can have your own garden and raise your own chickens, go for it! I do understand that for the majority of us that's impossible. In that case, connect with the farmer. It's just as important to have "a farmer" as it is to have a family doctor, if not more. If you get your food from local small farmers who grow food (plants and animals) according to the old traditional farming techniques, free of synthetic fertilizers and pesticides, insecticides, or herbicides, then chances are you're getting good quality food.

As much as possible, eat locally grown and raised foods. Eat seasonal. Keep away from genetically engineered foods. By eating organic whole foods, you will eliminate a great percentage of genetically engineered foods.

When it comes to plants, it's important to buy them organic. If that's not possible, keep in mind the Dirty Dozen and the Clean 15 lists.

The Environmental Working Group (EWG) releases a yearly list of crops that, when grown conventionally, have the greatest pesticide retention. These make the dirty dozen list. You can download their app to your smartphone or get the downloadable wallet size card directly from their site.

Below is the Dirty Dozen plus list and the Clean 15. I highly recommend to do your best to make an effort to purchase the foods on the Dirty Dozen in organic form.

Dirty Dozen, EWG's 2017 Shopper's Guide to Pesticides in Produce™ [41]

Dirty Dozen Plus	Clean 15
strawberries	sweet corn
spinach	avocados
nectarines	pineapples
apples	cabbage
peaches	onions
pears	sweet peas (frozen)
cherries	papayas
grapes	asparagus
celery	mangos
tomatoes	eggplant
sweet bell peppers	honeydew melon
potatoes	kiwi
hot peppers	cantaloupe
	cauliflower
	grapefruit

*Copyright © Environmental Working Group, www.ewg.org. Reproduced with permission.

When it comes to animal food, it is just as important to select good quality. I talked about this in the Protein 101 section; however, I will reinforce it here as well. Find small farmers that raise the animals out on the pasture, free range, and allow them to eat grass and be exposed to sun. The quality of their meat, eggs and fat is far superior to those that are raised in confinement. Something else to keep in mind is that animals, just like us, store toxins in the adipose tissue. Animals that are fed growth hormones, antibiotics, steroid drugs, etc., store those pollutants their fat tissue. When we consume such animal products, it increases the toxic overload of our body and it has a negative impact on our health.[47]

Beauty products and your health

Toxic accumulation leads to disease and impairs your ability to heal. Eating organic foods, non-GMO, grass fed animal products and "clean," wild caught fish is part of any healing protocol. This is not only due to better nutrient composition of those foods, but due to the fact that they come with a less toxic load.

What else from the environment contributes to the toxic overload that affects our body?

The water, the air, as well as the products that we use to clean our home and clothes with; cookware and storage containers as well as personal care and beauty products, all can contribute to the toxicity of the body and ill health. When it comes to personal care products we should be twice as careful.

Our skin is the largest organ. What we put on our skin is absorbed directly into the bloodstream and it bypasses the liver filtration. When we ingest something orally, food or drinks, the toxins that may be present in those are sent from the gut to the liver first. The liver metabolizes nutrients, drugs, toxins and, by doing this, helps eliminate some or most of the toxins we ingest. However, when we apply something on our skin, it gets absorbed directly into the systemic circulation; it doesn't get to the liver. Therefore, if it is toxic, it won't be cleared away. The toxins absorbed from personal care products and laundry products can cause more harm even than those ingested through food and water.

These are environmental factors we have full control over. We can choose to use less harmful products, which support healing. Drink clean (filtered) water; breath clean (filtered) air; use safe, non-toxic, biodegradable household cleaners; and apply on your skin only the beauty products you are also willing to eat. That is my philosophy.

In the resources section, you will come across few such beauty products.

PART 6:

HOW WE HEAL BEYOND FOOD

This section of the book is a brief look at other lifestyle factors that contribute to one's health, healing and better overall life. I will touch the surface of such factors as sleep, stress, and movement.

Healing requires many elements aside from food. No Lego® is built by using only one giant piece. Same goes for our health. It wouldn't be fair if I would say all you need to do to get healthy is to "fix" what you eat. No, it's so much more than that. In fact, there are many books written on each one of these factors.

My intent here is not to exhaust the list of the elements that contribute to health, nor to go deep into how they work. My intention is to review a few, to raise your awareness about their importance, and from here you can see which one you may be missing or you need to devote your attention to more.

6.1 MOVEMENT AND EXERCISE

They seem to be one and the same thing, but they are not. There is a distinct difference between movement and exercise. Nevertheless, they are both important in health and healing.

One day, I had this epiphany: *The reason we need to exercise today is because habitual movement is lost from our life.* If we look at how our ancestors lived, or if we observe one of the tribes that still live today in isolation from the modern "civilized" world, we can see that the only reason we need to exercise today (as in planned physical activity, like running, weight lifting, gym workout, CrossFit, etc.) is simply because habitual movement (such as walking for miles to migrate to better living places, running to catch prey, digging for roots, climbing trees, building shelters) is almost entirely gone from our lives.

Let me define movement:

Movement is the opposite of stagnation or prolonged inaction (prolonged sitting, standing or lying down). Often, people refer to movement as habitual movement or activities of daily living. Think of walking, climbing, bending, and reaching out, up or sideways. All of these motions are used when we perform daily tasks, such as cleaning, gardening, going places or carrying things.

A lifestyle that includes lots of habitual movement is an active one. Today, we have lost many of these movements, mainly because we are "blessed" with so many energy saving devices. Cars, planes, elevators, escalators, drive-thru, remote controls, dishwashers, washer and dryers are just some examples of the many modern day devices that make our life easier, but at the same time make it so that we don't have to move.

Although we live in a fast paced society, we're sitting a lot, or not moving nearly enough to support the health and function of our body. For the majority of us, our jobs require sitting. Our modern life goes like this: sitting at a desk sitting while driving, sitting while operating a machine, sitting or standing on a bus or train, and sitting or lying down when we get home and have downtime. Even writing this book required a lot of sitting or standing up at my desk.

If we were to contrast this with how our ancestors lived, we can see that there's a huge difference in their lifestyle and ours, as their lifestyle involved tremendous use of the human body; they walked a lot, they bent, they ran, they climbed.

I'm talking about this not to emphasize the calories in and calories out. I don't endorse the theory "we eat more, we don't move enough therefore we are gaining weight." No. I'm talking about movement from a functional perspective; from a health point of view.

When you move your body the way it was intended, you maintain functionality, as in joint mobility, muscle and ligament flexibility, agility and balance. You maintain your independence as you age.

Another factor that comes into play when we talk about prolonged sitting or standing is the effect gravity has on our body. This wonderful force that we have here on Earth has a miraculous effect on our body, if we use it. What do I mean by "if we use it?"

We know from research done on astronauts in space that the human body in the absence of gravity deteriorates. Structural and functional changes take place. The immune system's function is affected. Vision, cardiovascular health, muscles and bones suffer losses. Research performed on bedridden people show similar degenerative processes take place in the human body while in a state of prolonged sitting or lying down. Inactivity in the presence of gravity has the same deteriorating effects on the human body as the absence of gravity does on the astronauts when they spend time in space. Dr. Joan Vernikos, PhD has researched this topic and she wrote a brilliant book, "Sitting Kills, Moving Heals." I highly recommend reading her book.

The two important elements here are gravity and movement, or the absence of it. Together, they form a good partnership; in fact, a perfect marriage.

Movement + Gravity = Health

Inactivity + Gravity = Disease

Another way I like to say it is if we don't "wrestle" with the gravity it "pulls us down."

So what should you do, to prevent gravity from playing its negative effect on your body?

Begin by doing an activity inventory. Look at a 24-hour day; how much of your time is spent in prolonged sitting, standing or lying down? If you have acquired a "movement deficit," even if you engage in 1 hour of planned exercise a day every day, it's simply not enough to compensate for the lack of movement during the other 20 plus hours.

To prevent this, you need to make a conscious effort to incorporate more movement into your life. Walk more, carry things, climb up the stairs, dance, bend to pick up things, or sweep and mop the floor. Do things that get your body moving. If you get to move more outdoors, that's even better!

A strategy I personally use, and recommended to all of my clients in order to add movement to a long work day in front of the computer, is to set a timer for a 30 minute work interval, followed by a 2 minute work break. During the 2 minute break, you can stand up and do some exercises (squats, lunges, push-ups, mini jumps, get on a rebounder, do stairs, use resistance bands or light weight for the upper body muscles). It is particularly beneficial if you engage your body in movements that involve big muscles and go against gravity (up, down and sideways).

The 30:2 rule of movement will transform your mind and body, and it will in crease your productivity too.

Believe it or not, this 2 minute exercise session every 30 minutes actually increases your muscle tone, flexibility, strength and even cardiovascular fitness, especially if you choose to add High Intensity Interval Training.

Moving is not only good for your physical body, but for your energetic body, as well. It helps you move your energy around. The more you sit (don't move), the more your energy stagnates—your creative energy, your productivity energy, your healing energy. The more you move, the more energy you generate, and the better you'll feel at all levels. You will have a better mood and actually get more things done.

What about planned exercise?

Exercise has many health benefits, and weight loss is not the main one. Is this surprising to you? Let me explain.

When you think that exercise is the element you need in order to lose weight, you set yourself up for failure. You are most likely to engage in an exercise regimen that is simply not sustainable long term (just like diets are not). As an example, you may engage in intense training sessions, running, biking, gym workouts, personal trainer sessions, etc. that are not sustainable long term. Often this is because they require too many hours of your already busy day, or they are scheduled at the most inconvenient times of the day (5 am, lunch break, 11 pm). At times, financially it can get difficult, as well. Not to mention, if an injury happens, you have to stop or reduce the time and intensity drastically.

The worst part of all, however, is thinking that you work out for one hour or more a day and now you can eat more, because you have "earned it."

You can't "earn your calories" with exercise, but you can "earn your shower."

In fact, that's one other reason I don't emphasize the caloric aspect of food. What happens with probably 90% of the people that have this approach to weight? They lose weight at first; but, since it is not a sustainable long term plan, they gain the weight back, and often gain more. Do you know why? They didn't quite learn how to maintain a healthy weight independent of them engaging in strenuous exercise. They didn't learn about the hormonal effect food has on the body. They are stuck on the calories in, calories out paradigm. Unfortunately, there is more to human metabolism then these energy exchanges. What I'm trying to convey here is to reframe the mindset from:

"exercise to eat" to "exercise to be fit."

Let's look at an example:

If you eat one slice of pepperoni pizza (approximately 4 oz.) and have only one beer (12 oz.) with it, that's approximately 450 cal. It takes about 2 hours of walking or 1 hour of cycling to "burn it off." That's a lot of exercise for a small meal, and how many people do you know that eat only one slice of pizza and drink only one beer?

If we were to exclude the real meaning of food (nourishment, healing, information, metabolic control) and reduce it to purely calories, you can see how difficult it would be to earn your calories with exercise.

Does this mean you shouldn't exercise? Not at all!

Exercise is the best antidepressant "drug" and mood enhancer out there. Exercise strengthens the heart and the entire cardiovascular system. It helps build strong bones and muscles. It helps you look and feel better in your own skin, both with clothes on as well as in bathing suits. It helps you maintain muscle mass as you age (and prevent age related sarcopenia). It helps improve balance, which is the most important aspect, aside from muscle mass, in age related fall prevention.

In conclusion, the mindset around exercise goes like this:

"Exercise to be fit. Don't exercise to eat! You will most likely overeat."

Now, let's talk about ways in which you can exercise.

There are many forms of exercise you can engage in that will give you all those mind and body health benefits. From strength training to HIIT to stretching, they can all enhance your life, health and beauty.

Personally, I'm a big fan of High Intensity Interval Training (HIIT) and for a good reason. HIIT, aside from improving cardiovascular fitness, helps increase the production of the Human Growth Hormone (HGH) and the brain derived neurotrophic factor (BDNF), two powerful anti-aging hormones which are important, especially as we grow older, as our body naturally produces less of them.

> *HIIT + Fasting + MRP = the most effective mind-body transformation strategy.*

So, how should you approach exercise? What role should it play in your life-body-health transformation journey?

I highly recommend not making changes in your exercise routine and your food regimen at the same time.

When you initiate such a big dietary change as we discussed in this book, MRP or GRP, your body needs time to adapt to it. Believe it or not, it is actually a stressful event for the body. Good stress, short term stress, but nevertheless, stress.

You need to master the food part first, and only after you feel comfortable with your eating plan, after it becomes second nature, and you don't need to think about it anymore, then you can think of spicing it up with some fun indoor and outdoor activities.

When it comes to planned activities (exercise), I think it is good to have a mix of resistance training (weight lifting or lifting your own body weight), aerobic/ cardiovascular (running, biking, swimming, kick boxing), stretching (yoga, Pilates, qi gong, tai chi), and the most effective of all forms of exercise, HIIT.

Let me explain how HIIT is done:

In a short period of time (as little as 4 minutes, 3 times a day, or as long as 20 minutes once a day) you can challenge your body in a good way and reap the benefits of both strength and aerobics all at once. There are many forms of HIIT. You can go to this link http://bit.ly/HIIT4YOU and see video demonstrations of it. The beauty of this training is that you go for a short duration at your max heart rate capacity, then you recover for a short duration and repeat this cycle several times.

> Always warm up for about 5 min at the beginning and cool down and stretch at the end.
>
> Tabata: [20 seconds sprint + 10 seconds recovery] X 8 = 4 min.
>
> You can do 1 Tabata 3 times a day.
>
> "Sprint 8": [30 seconds sprint + 90 seconds recovery] X 8 = 16 min.
>
> You can do "Sprint 8" 3 times a week.

At first this can seem very hard, but like anything else in life that's new, the more you practice, the better you get.

Some advantages of HIIT over traditional endurance exercise are:

- It's short duration. You can easily fit it into your busy schedule. Anyone can find 4 min three times a day.

- You can do it anywhere you are: at home, gym, park, beach, hotel, i you're traveling, etc.

- You can do it while walking: alternating fast walking with slow walking, running (sprint with run), pushups, squats, etc. It usually involves big muscles and moving your body against gravity.

Remember to check with your medical doctor before starting any exercise routine, including HIIT.

In conclusion, planned exercise is fabulous for its many health benefits, yet you should not see it as your weight loss tool. Food takes care of your weight. Engaging in habitual movement that involves big muscles going against gravity is far more important than 1 hour of exercise 5 times a week.

Move frequently and exercise regularly. Do it with joy and keep in mind what role each one plays in your overall health and happiness.

6.2 SLEEP AND STRESS

I don't think we can have a discussion about healing the mind and the body without talking about sleep. Nightly sleep is crucial for regular repairs and rejuvenation, as well as for healing. Sleep is like a built-in reset system our body has. From brain function to detox and weight loss, all are impacted by the quality and the amount of sleep we get.

Living in the 21st century in industrialized countries not only affects what we eat and how we move, but also affects our sleep. It used to be that we went to sleep with the sun set and got up with the sun rise. It is a natural circadian rhythm that our body is biologically programed to follow. Now, we have electricity and that changes the scenario quite a bit. It gives us longer days (with artificial light on at night) and shorter nights. If we add to that the amount of time we spend in front of the blue light screens (from phones, to tablets and TV), I'm am not surprised that so many of us today struggle with poor quality sleep and simply can't get enough good sleep.

Sleep deprivation is quite the norm, and it comes at a high health, weight and productivity cost. When we add to all of these the stress of our fast-paced lives, the picture gets even worse.

Stress is a normal response of our body to a threat; a built in survival mechanism.

"The tiger is chasing you or your family. You respond appropriately; you are able to generate a burst of energy to power up your brain and muscles to save yourself or your loved ones from the life-threatening event." It's the sympathetic nervous system's response to stress: a flight or fight reaction. This is an immediate acute stress response, facilitated by an elevation in adrenaline and cortisol, which induces physiological responses that allow us to fight and escape the dangerous situation.

What are some of the physical manifestations of stress? Sudden increase in blood glucose, due to the liver's excess glucose production, heart rate goes up, blood starts to pump harder to supply enough oxygen and glucose to the working muscles, while functions such as digestion will be significantly slowed down.

Fortunately, our lives today don't encounter too many life or death emergency situations. However, our lives are more often under a chronic low-grade stress, which leads to a low-grade stress response, and keeps us with chronically elevated levels of cortisol and adrenalin. What does that mean for us?

It means chronically elevated blood sugar, or difficulty maintaining stable blood sugar; increased heart rate and blood pressure; and chronic low-grade inflammation.

The cycle of ill health gets bigger and stronger, and it leads to more and more chronic diseases.

The best analogy I can use to illustrate this is the transformation of a tropical storm into a category 5 hurricane. As it travels through the ocean, if it has the right environmental conditions, the tropical storm keeps gaining strength until it becomes a hurricane. Same goes for our body: if the right environmental conditions are present (poor food, lack of sleep, stress, lack of movement, lack of fresh air and clean water, insufficient nature interaction, lack of social integration, exposure to drugs, etc.), the body gets weaker and, eventually, starts to break down. That is when disease sets in.

The equivalent of the hurricane for the human body is the manifestation of various chronic diseases.

Does this look familiar? *You had a poor night of sleep and got up late, had to rush out of the house, grabbed a drive thru coffee and a doughnut. Now, you are stuck in traffic, are late to work, and you are behind with your project. Your boss calls you to his office. You get a call from school because your kids are sick, and you need to take time off to take them to the doctor. It's 5 pm and you realized you still need to go get groceries and cook. You forgot to pick up the clothes from the dry cleaner and still need to finish up laundry.*

That's the fast-paced life most of us live today. That's what soaks our body in stress hormones. That's chronic low-grade stress.

What are you to do? Change what you have control over! Start with sleep.

Tips for a better sleep:

- Prioritize your sleep.

- Develop a personal nighttime ritual. Set up a bed time goal and wake up goal. Do that every day, including weekends.

Some things to include into your nighttime ritual to assure better sleep quality are:

- Reduce exposure to blue light.

  o Use phone and computer apps that filter out the blue light. For example, for the computer you can use f.lux.

  o Use orange glasses (blue blockers) to filter out the blue light. You can get those through an optometrist office.

  o Set your phone to "night-time" mode to reduce its blue light.

- Expose your eyes and your skin daily to sunlight.

- Avoid screen time 2-3 hours before your set bed time.

- Stop eating and drinking about 2-3 hours before your set bed time.

- Journal your day's wins and gratitude. Focus on the blessings in your life.

- Do a "brain dump" on paper with all the things you have in your mind that need to be taken care of the next day or that week.

- Have a relaxing bath with candles and relaxing music. Add to the water Epsom salt, lavender oil, etc.

- Read a book.

- Listen to a guided meditation.

- Do a visualization exercise.

Tips for managing chronic stress:

- Become a master at prioritizing things in your day.

- Learn to delegate and ask for help.

- Learn to receive help.

- Embrace the mantra *"progress before perfection."*

- Learn when you need to say no and say it.

- Avoid getting upset about things you have no control over.

- Practice deep, nasal breathing, especially if you feel anxious.

- Make a practice of walking outdoors and being in nature. If possible, do it barefoot.

- Practice yoga, tai chi, qi gong.

- Partake in meditation, visualization, or journaling.

These are only a few suggestions. Find what works for you and give those aspects of life just as high of a priority as you give food.

Another suggestion is, when you start the healing journey and set your goals, think of the best way to prioritize all the many aspects of your life in which you'll need to make adjustments.

Prioritize your:

- food

- movement

- sleep

- stress

- spirituality/mindset

- "me"/fun time

6.3 NATURE THERAPY

I believe the best therapy for the human mind and body is being out in nature. As always, I like to imagine how our ancestors lived. They were in nature and part of nature. Today, we are disconnected from nature; we are almost fighting against our own home.

I'd like to invite you to spend more time in nature, under the sun and even in the rain. Walk, climb, swim, have a picnic or camp. Be away from electricity, TV, cell phones, hot showers and climate controlled rooms. Get together with family and friends around a campfire and just talk, play games, or share stories.

There is healing and strengthening in doing that.

Being barefoot in contact with the Earth has powerful health benefits. Some may argue there is not enough scientific evidence to back up this statement. I'll be honest: I don't need a scientific study to tell me that spending time out in nature and being barefoot in direct contact with the Earth is good for me. I can feel it. Every time I spend time at the beach or in a park, I feel incredible. It has a mind and body boosting effect.

There is a scientific explanation to why we feel that way: the earth sends its negative charge into the human body; this negative charge acts as a powerful antioxidant and aids in healing. This is known as "grounding" or "earthing." A good book to read on this subject is "Earthing: The Most Important Health Discovery Ever?" by C. Ober, S. Sinatra, MD, and M. Zucker.

The earth is a big charger that we all need to plug ourselves into to keep ourselves functioning optimally. We are tiny electric human devices that need to be periodically charged, otherwise we can't function. The best way for us to recharge is to simply be in contact with the earth, barefooted. Find safe ways to walk barefoot on the earth (beach, grass, even cement). Keep in mind, to get the negative charge of the earth, you need to be on a material that is a good electricity conductor. Rubber, wood, asphalt, plastic and tar are not. Earth (beach, grass, dirt), water, cement and leather are.

Aside from the negative charge from the earth, we get so many benefits from being out in nature; from sun to microbes, we get them all. A good exchange of microbes between us and the environment happens especially when we put our hands in dirt and get really close to it. The best way to do that is to garden. I believe the ultimate healing and anti-inflammatory activity is gardening. It's done outdoors, provides a good dose of sun, earth/dirt and water; it facilitates a good exchange of microbes between us and the earth. It's also a form of creative art and usually it involves other people, so it strengthens human inter-action, and at the end of it all, it generates real whole foods.

Sun and natural light exposure are crucial elements of health and healing, and they stretch their health benefits beyond vitamin D and melatonin production. Add sensible sun exposure to your life and healing journey. Expose your skin to sun, early in the morning and later in the evening, and allow your body to respond with melanin (that's when your skin gets brown and you get a nice A suntan). A suntan offers natural built-in sun protection; the tanner you are, the less you will burn. You'll be able to enjoy the full spectrum of benefits associat-ed with sunlight and outdoor activities.

Of course, I do not suggest you stay in the sun in the middle of the day. That time of the day is for siesta under the shade of a tree, or in a nice cool room. A suntan is safe, sunburn is not.

We may not always have a clear explanation as to how something works or why we do things a certain way, but eventually modern day science comes with an explanation for it, and that makes us feel good; it validates our actions. How-ever, we don't always have to wait for modern science to confirm or explain the obvious. Sometimes, we just have to trust that our inner wisdom finds the solution to our problems. Food, Movement, Sleep, Nature, Earth, Sun, are all elements of the healing journey.

PART 7: RESOURCES

7.1 Metabolic Superfoods

The term superfood is used a lot. The food industry knows its power. That's why you will see it on many exotic foods, such as goji berries, acai berries and cacao nibs.

My intention here in attaching the term superfood to these everyday foods is simply to indicate that these are foods that have a high nutritional value and can support your body to heal, whether you are using the MR or the GR protocol.

Avocados.

They are a nutrient dense food, containing vitamins and minerals such as pantothenic acid, vitamin K, copper, folate, vitamin B6, potassium, magnesium, vitamin E, and vitamin C. They are also an excellent source of fat (monounsaturated fats). They are creamy, versatile and wonderfully delicious! Although avocado is classified as a fruit, most of its carbohydrate content is fiber, so it is a low Net Carb fruit or a non-insulinogenic food. Avocado is a great source of potassium, which becomes particularly important when following the low carb lifestyle.

Most of the calories of avocado come from fat (21X9=189 - out of 227). Good fats, such as those found in avocadoes and nuts, are to be embraced wholeheartedly. Here are some reasons why avocados should find their way onto your plate: [51]

- The fat in avocado aids in absorption of fat-soluble vitamins such as beta carotene and vitamins A, D, E and K, as they cannot be absorbed without fat. This is why avocado makes a great addition to any salad;

- It only has 3 g of NC. There are approximately 12 g of carbs in 1 Hass avocado; however, if we subtract the fiber (9 grams), we are left with 3 g of Net Carbs;

- In just one avocado, there is about 689 mg of potassium. This makes avocados a great food for athletes and active people, as well as if you are following the MR or GR protocols;

- Avocado is rich in folate. This vitamin is important in the production and maintenance of new cells. It is especially important during pregnancy and infancy when cells are rapidly developing and growing. Folate is also needed in adults and children for the production of red blood cells and to prevent anemia; [54]

- A good source of vitamin E, avocados helps boost the immune system. This vitamin is also used to help cells communicate and interact with each other and carry out many important functions within the body.

Now that you know a little bit more about this amazing superfood, here are some ways you can start adding it into your diet:

- Add it as a garnish or on the side of almost any meal. I love eating it with eggs, on a salad, or even just slicing it up with some tomato, a little salt and pepper and drizzling it with olive oil!

- By itself as a snack. Cut it in half, remove the pit and scoop it up with a spoon.

- Homemade guacamole: you can use veggies such as celery, bell peppers, or cucumbers instead of tortilla chips, or use it as a "sauce" for any main course.

- Blend it in a smoothie. You can't even taste it! It just makes your smoothie more thick, creamy, and delicious! The added fat will slow the absorption of sugar from fruits into your bloodstream and keep you feeling full for a longer period of time.

How to pick and store avocados

Before cutting open an avocado, make sure it is ripe. The skin is mostly all brown and they are slightly squishy. The stem at the top of the avocado will easily come off and leave a golden spot if already ripe. Hint, ripe fruits and vegetables are more easily digested and their nutrients are more bioavailable (more effectively absorbed).

If the avocados are green and hard when you purchase them, leave them on the kitchen counter to ripen in a brown paper bag. When they are ripe and ready, you can store them in brown paper bags inside the refrigerator and they will last for days, even weeks.

Versatile ways to use avocados

Aside from eating them, you can use avocados to make beauty products. Here's a recipe I make from time to time to make my skin more supple:

- Take ¼ avocado, add few drops of lemon juice, 1 tsp. olive oil, ¼ tsp. clay and ¼ tsp. charcoal.

- Mix all the ingredients well to form a paste.

- Apply it to your face, neck and chest, in a thin layer.

- Lay down and listen to relaxing music for 15-30 min.

- Then, wash it off.

Avocado oil makes a great body oil and skin moisturizer. I recommend buying it from the cooking aisle, not from the beauty products section.

Almonds.

Almonds are packed with many vitamins and minerals including magnesium, phosphorus, calcium, vitamin E, iron, zinc, copper, niacin, selenium, and copper.[51] Compared with all other nuts, almonds are the most nutrient dense. However, most nuts do share a lot of the same nutrient composition.

Almonds are not the only nut to incorporate into your diet. Walnuts, pine nuts, macadamia nuts, hemp seeds, and pecans are all low carb nuts and can easily be incorporated into your food plan.

For a side by side nuts and seeds comparison see Table 1 on page 294.

Here, I'll focus on almonds, but remember all nuts are good, so pick those you love the most and add them to your diet.

- Most of the carbohydrates found in almonds are in the form of fiber. In 1 oz., there are 3.3 g of fiber out of a total of 5.6 g. This makes it a great food to eat when following a low carb diet, providing only 2.3 g of net carbs per 1 oz. serving;

- Almonds are also a great source of plant-based protein. There are 6 g in just 1 oz. This, combined with the amount of fat they contain, will help to control blood sugar levels and keep you feeling full for longer. They are a great snack, especially when you are first transitioning to the MRF or GRP (if tolerated);

- The fats in almonds (14 g of fat in 1 oz. serving) are mostly monoun saturated and are considered to have cardiovascular protective benefits. Almonds also contain a small amount of the linolenic (omega-3) fatty acids which helps control inflammation;

• Almonds are rich in antioxidants, vitamin A and glutathione. Glutathione is the most important antioxidant your body makes and almonds help your body to produce more of it;

• They are a good source of potassium (206 mg per 1 oz. serving).

How to incorporate almonds and nuts into your diet?

You may be thinking, "Wow, almonds really are a super-food! I need to start adding them into my diet, but plain raw almonds are just so boring." Luckily for you, there are many other ways to add almonds into your diet that will leave your taste buds begging for more! Here are some examples:

• Almond butter: try spreading it on a cucumber or zucchini, blending it in a smoothie, or just digging into the jar for a big 'ol spoonful. That's how I do it! Any nut or seed butter is delicious and makes for a quick snack. I also like to use almond butter to make a pizza crust.

• Almond milk (preferably homemade to avoid all the gums added to store bought almond milk): you can follow the same recipe as for the pine nut-hemp milk, but you will need to strain the milk through a nut bag or cheesecloth. That's the reason I don't make almond milk and I stick with macadamia, pine nuts, hemp seeds and cashew milk, or a blend of those; they are less fibrous, so there is no need to strain them.

• Almond flour: use as a substitution for grain flours in baking and other cooking. This is a good low carb option to use when cooking. You can even make your own by pulsing raw almonds in the food processor or blending until they are ground up and grainy.

Almonds are a great snack to have on the go or when you are in a rush. I like to grab a handful of mixed nuts to eat as a snack to hold me over until my next meal. TIP: For better digestion and absorption of nutrients from nuts, it is best to soak raw nuts including almonds overnight and then dehydrate them at low temperature before eating them. High temperatures from roasting nuts denatures and breaks down their delicate fats. For a video recipe on how to prep nuts for better digestion, please go to https://www.mihaelatelecan.com/nuts-digestible/.

Buying and Storing Tips

- Almonds can be bought at almost any grocery store. Most grocery stores have them packaged, but if you go to a health store, you can probably find them in a bulk bin. If you live near a Costco, that is also a great place to buy them in larger bags for a reasonable price. Almonds can also be bought online if you can't find exactly what you are looking for in any store.

- I recommend storing all nuts and seeds in the freezer, as their fats can easily go rancid if stored at room temperature. Ideally, we should buy all nuts in their hard shell, take them out of the shell only when ready to reactivate them and consume them rapidly after that. Since that is less likely to happen, find a store that sells a lot. They are always fresh and you can keep them in your freezer until you are ready to consume them.

Cabbage (and its family).

These are also known as cruciferous or brassica vegetables. Here are some examples of brassica foods:

- broccoli, broccoli rabe, cauliflower, all types of cabbage, brussels sprouts, kale, collards, turnips, turnip and mustard greens, arugula, watercress, bok choy, Chinese cabbage, kohlrabi, radishes, and daikon.

They all have the same incredible health benefits, and can help keep your body healthy, thriving, and full of energy.

- They are high volume, low carb foods, with high water and fiber content;

- The true superfood-nutritional value of the brassica foods comes from the powerful sulfur-containing compounds known as glucosinolate.[33] Those compounds give the spicy and or bitter taste of the crucifer ous vegetables. During chopping or chewing of brassica vegetables, the glucosinolates compounds are converted by an enzyme (myrosinase) present in the plant's cell walls into biologically active compounds like indoles and isothiocyanates. These are known as organosulfur compounds and are responsible for the many health benefits of brassica foods, from detoxification, to cancer prevention, to reduced inflammation, to collagen synthesis;[33]

• They've been shown to help protect the brain and the body from excessive inflammation by ramping up the production of glutathione, reducing markers for degenerative damage in the nervous system, and slowing or even reversing age-related declines in brain function and cognitive performance;[33]

• Regular, long term consumption of these vegetables have been shown to reduce the risk of heart disease and many cancers (colorectal, lung, breast, and prostate), support detoxification, stimulate the immune system, slow down cognitive decline and support longevity.[51]

Cooking tips to maximize health gains

• When cooking with brassica vegetables, it is best to cut them and let them sit for at least 5 minutes before you cook or eat them, just like you would with garlic or onions. This allows them to react with oxygen and activate the antioxidant compounds. It also allows the myrosinase to breakdown the glucosinolates into those active phytonutrients. Exposure to oxygen will also help reduce the sulfuric smell they give off when you cook them;

• Many people with thyroid dysfunction avoid brassica foods due to their goitrogenic compounds. However, when cooked or fermented, some of the goitrogenic compounds are lost; hence, they can be enjoyed in small amounts. Goitrogenic compounds have been found to interfere with the thyroid hormone synthesis and it affects people with hypothyroidism, especially if consumed raw and in large amounts;

• Brassica vegetables, and cabbage in particular, have the incredible

ability to turn into another amazing superfood: fermented vegetables—
the queen of all fermented vegetables being sauerkraut;

• Fermented vegetables not only provide you with many beneficial microorganisms, they also give you the prebiotic-fiber and the nutrients in
a more bioavailable form. The friendly microbes are literally unlocking
many of the micronutrients trapped inside the cell walls of the plants
and making them more bio-available (they pre-digest for us).

Berries.

The dark blueish/purple color of blueberries and blackberries, and the bright
red and pink of strawberries, raspberries and goji berries are where their powerful antioxidant properties come from.

The pigments that give the vibrant colors we see in the "rainbow"
of vegetables and fruits are the powerful antioxidants and phytonutrients. They make plants powerful cleanser, anti-oxidant and anti-inflammatory foods. The darker the color the stronger the antioxidant
power of the plant. Always, when you eat plant food focus on getting
a great variety of colors: "eat the rainbow." The active compounds
responsible for the many health benefits of berries are called flavo-
noids.[33]

From all the berries out there, most of the research has been done on blueberries. It shows that they improve memory, cognitive function, and blood flow to
the brain. They also help to protect against damage from free radicals.

All berries, not just blueberries, are a great brain food. When it comes to berries and their glycemic impact or insulinogenic effect, there is great individua
variability. My suggestion is to test your blood sugar before you eat berries as
well as after you eat them. Based on your glycemic response to them, you'l
know which ones you can eat and in what amount.

Purchasing tips:

- When purchasing berries, it is very important to purchase them organic. Unfortunately, berries are on the Dirty Dozen list. When grown conventionally and sprayed with pesticides, herbicides, insecticides, etc., the chemicals are absorbed into the fruit and you are then putting those harmful chemicals into your body. This takes away from the "super" qualities of the berries.

- Buying frozen, organic berries is also a great way to keep berries in your house all year long, even outside of their growing season. Look for bags of frozen berries that have nothing added to them. These are great for adding in green-smoothies, yogurt, or just eating plain. Frozen berries are sometimes even better than fresh ones, because they are at their prime ripeness when they are picked and immediately frozen. They actually hold their nutritional content pretty well when frozen, so you are not missing out on any goodness!

Most grocery stores carry berries both fresh and frozen. Again Costco is a great place to get organic, sometimes fresh and always frozen, berries.

For a quick look at different berries and their NC, refer to Table 2 on page 295.

Coconut oil.

There are countless reasons to love coconut and its oil. It is very versatile; it can be used from the kitchen, to the bathroom (makes a great beauty product), and even to the bedroom as the best lubricant ever. Coconut oil is really an incredible food. Let's see what coconut oil is and what makes it so special:

- Coconut oil is a tropical fat extracted from the coconut;

- Most of the fat in coconut oil is saturated fat; however, what makes coconut oil special as a saturated fat is the length of the fatty acids. About two thirds of the fatty acids in coconut oil are medium-chain fatty acids (MCFAs).[51] These types of fatty acids produce a whole host of health benefits. In fact, coconut oil is nature's richest source of these healthy MCTs. What makes coconut oil a superfood is the high concentration of medium chain triglycerides (MCTs).

When you follow a low carbohydrate diet and you burn fat for fuel, coconut oil becomes prime real estate.

Is it coconut oil or coconut butter?

You may feel confused about this. What makes coconut oil turn into butter? The short answer is the temperature:

- Liquid (oil) at 75°F (25°C) or above; and

- Solid (butter) at any temperature below 75°F (25°C).

If you ever heard anyone calling it coconut "butter," they are just referring to the solid form of coconut oil; it is the same product.

Other ways to use coconut oil

- It can be used as a full body moisturizer (add few drops of essential oils to it like lavender or frankincense for additional benefits and perfume);

- You can apply it on your hair if you have dry hair or to enhance curls;

- It is great for oil pulling (old method of cleaning the teeth and detoxing the oral cavity). Take a tablespoon of coconut oil in your mouth and swish it gently for 15 minutes. At the end of the 15 minutes discard the oil;

- It's a great base for toothpaste and deodorants.

Buying and storing coconut oil

When buying coconut oil, it is very important to look for:

- organic, because conventionally grown coconuts are highly sprayed with pesticides, fertilizers, and other toxins that you do not want to be putting into your body;

- unrefined and cold pressed;

- preferably non-GMO coconut oil;

• although I mentioned before that coconut oil is not as easily dam-aged by light or heat as other oils are, it is still best to store it in a cool dark place, like inside a cabinet;

• glass containers, however, should you buy it in a plastic container, make sure it is BPA free, as it is a safer material than regular plastic.

Chia seeds.

The chia plant (Salvia hispanica) is native to central and southern Mexico and Guatemala. It belongs to the mint family.[53] The seeds of this plant have been used by Latin Americans and Southwest American Indians for centuries as a staple food source, for sustenance during endurance contests and to treat constipation. Today, you can find chia seeds on the shelf in most supermarkets all over the world.

So, what's the hype about chia seeds and should you buy into it? The hype is backed up by the multiple health benefits and the rich nutritional composition of these black, tiny seeds.

• Chia seeds are rich in antioxidants, phytonutrients, fiber, omega-3 fatty acids and are a complete protein (they contains all the 9 essential amino acids);

• Those tiny seeds are a great source of dietary fiber, mostly soluble fiber;

• If we look at the carbs in chia seeds, in 1 oz. (28 g) we find 12.4 g of total carbohydrates and 10.7 g of fiber. That means it only has 1.7 g NC. It is great to add chia to your diet to increase fiber intake, especially if you have a tendency towards constipation. Check the recipes section, as I share a very yummy chia pudding recipe;

• Most people can tolerate chia seeds better than flax seeds. They cause less gastric distress (gas, bloating, pain);

• Most of the fats in chia are polyunsaturated (7 g out of 9 g). Due to its fatty acid composition (40% omega-6 fats and 30% omega-3 fats), it is considered an anti-inflammatory and heart healthy food, with an opti-mal ratio of omega-6 to omega-3 fats;

- It's a good source of vegetable protein (4 g per oz.), containing all the 9 essential amino acids. If you are a plant eater, you've got to love chia;

- Great source of potassium, calcium and iron, which makes it a great sports recovery food;

- Makes a great egg substitute in recipes. 2 tsp. ground chia seeds mixed with 3 tbsp. boiling water, let it sit for 5 min, then use in any recipe instead of 1 egg.

Grass fed meat, eggs and organ meats.

When we talk about animal food, quality is more important than quantity. Throughout the book, I talked about the importance of getting your animal products from grass-fed, pasture raised animals. Here I want to emphasize the nutrient density.

Animal foods are your most nutrient dense foods. But not all animal products provide the same nutrient density. The most nutrient dense are the organ meats and not the cuts of muscle meats. Animal foods supply us with all the vitamins we need. There are two vitamins we can't get from animal foods in considerable amounts: vitamin C and vitamin K1. These two are best acquired by consuming vegetables and fruits. [54] All the rest are found in animal foods or are produced by the gut flora—another reason to have a well-balanced gut microbiome. Evolutionarily it makes sense; our ancestors didn't always have access to plant foods, hence the gut microbes produced the vitamins that were not supplied by the food.

Best sources of nutrient dense animal foods are:

Eggs and organ meats (liver, heart, kidneys, lungs, gizzards and tongue).[54]

o These are an excellent source of all the vitamins like B1, B5, B2, Biotin folic acid, and Vitamin D3 and K2;

o They are a great source of iron and zinc, as well as coenzyme Q10; and o The richest food source of CoQ10 is the heart. CoQ10 is crucial for energy production. In fact, the heart muscle has the highest demand for it.

Note: If you are taking statin drugs to lower your cholesterol, keep in mind that they also block your body's ability to produce CoQ10, so it may be a good idea not only to eat more hearts, but to also supplement with CoQ10.

Bones, bone marrow and joints (feet, necks, tails, and wings).

These are a staple to making the most gut and immune healing meal: "the meat and bone stock."

The meat/bone stock is one of the richest sources of amino acids, fatty acids and minerals, all important nutrients for healing the gut and the body. You are probably asking, where will you find grass fed bones and organ meats?

A good resource is Weston A Price Foundation. On their website, you will find a directory of farms that you can trust, as they are raising animals providing the best conditions for the animal as well as for the environment; hence, for all of us. Visit https://www.westonaprice.org/find-nutrient-dense-foods/.

Seaweed.

I know, you're probably thinking "Seaweed? Isn't that the stuff floating around in the ocean?" Well, actually yes, it is! But there are many different kinds of seaweed: some that we eat and some that we don't. So why is seaweed a superfood and how do we eat it? The term seaweed refers to several species of macroscopic, multicellular marine algae. Seaweed has a long culinary history in many Asian countries, but it has become a very popular food in all parts of the world.

You are most likely to find seaweed used to wrap up sushi, in miso soup, or made into seaweed salad. However, there are also many other ways to utilize this extremely nutrient dense and tasty food in your everyday life. As I mentioned before, there are a few types of seaweed that we regularly eat. Here are few of the most common ones:

- Dulse flakes are raw flakes of seaweed that can be added to salads, soups, or even smoothies for some extra nutrients;

- Kombu looks like a hard stick of plastic, but when you put it in water, stock, or soups, it softens up, and allows many minerals and nutrients to leach into your food. This is the kind of seaweed that you normally will find in miso soup. You can add kombu when you make a meat/bone stock to increase the mineral load of the stock, and discard it at the end;

- Nori is the type of seaweed that is usually wrapped around your sushi;

- You can buy toasted seaweed snacks at the grocery store that are a fun snack to eat and kids love them too!

A few reasons to add seaweeds to your plate:

- Seaweed (kelp, kombu, and arame) is one of the best sources of iodine, a mineral that is used in all parts of your body, but is primarily used by the thyroid to produce the thyroid hormones;[54]

- Seaweed also provides your body with all the necessary nutrients to promote mitochondrial function. Remember, that mitochondria are organelles inside our cells that are responsible for converting food into energy. Minerals and vitamins in seaweed enhance this process, allowing your body to get the most energy out of the food we eat;

- Seaweed has high levels of selenium, which promotes proper immune function;

- The high levels of magnesium in seaweed promote good nerve and muscle function, and aid in the metabolism of carbohydrates;

- Seaweed (hijiki, arame, and wakame) also has about ten times as much calcium as other vegetables;[55]

- Wakame, kombu and nori are a good source of soluble fiber. [55]

As you can see, seaweeds are packed with minerals, and are a super-food. Unfortunately, seaweed is also one of the harder foods to digest. However, having a strong and healthy gut allows for the best digestion and most absorption of nutrients, including those from seaweed.

Soaking helps digest seaweeds. The longer you soak them, the easier they are to digest. You can also use the soaking water to make soup. This concludes the everyday super foods section. Of course, there are more superfoods than what I covered here; we could fill up another book with them. I picked the ones that I think are the most powerful and are a good fit for anyone following a low carb, high fat metabolic or gut reset protocol.

7.2 Nuts & Seeds, Fruits and Cheese: Macronutrients at A Glance

Table 1: Selected Nuts & Seeds

Nut/seed 1 oz.	Total Carbs g	Fiber g	Net Carbs g	Protein g	Fat g	Energy Calories
Almonds	5.6	3.3	2.3	6	14	164
Brazil Nut	3.3	2.1	3.2	4	19	187
Cashews	8.6	0.9	7.7	5	12	157
Chia Seed	11.9	9.8	2.1	5	9	138
Coconut	4.3	2.6	1.7	0.9	10	100
Flax Seed	8.2	7.7	0.5	5	12	151
Hazlenut	4.7	2.6	2.1	4	17	178
Hemp seed	7.8	7.8	0	7	10	149
Macadamia	3.9	2.4	1.5	2	22	204
Pecans	12.4	10.7	1.7	4	9	138
Pinenuts	5.5	3	2.5	3	17	178
Pistachio	7.8	2.9	4.9	6	13	159
Pumpkin Seed	4.2	1.8	2.4	9	14	163
Sesame Seeds	6.7	3.4	3.4	5	14	162
Sunflower Seeds	5.7	2.4	3.3	6	14	166
Walnuts	3.9	2	1.9	4	19	185

Table 2: Selected Fruits

Berries 1/2cup.	Total Carbs g	Fiber g	Net Carbs g	Protein g	Fat g	Energy Calories
Blackberries	6.9	3.8	3.1	1	0.4	31
Blueberries	10.7	1.8	8.9	0.5	0.2	42
Currants	8.6	3.8	4.8	0.8	0.2	35
Cranberries	6.1	2.3	3.8	0.2	0.1	23
Goji Berries	17.7	4.1	13.6	4	0.3	89
Grapefruit	12.3	1.8	10.5	0.9	0.2	48
Lemon	7.8	2.3	5.5	0.9	0.3	24
Lime	12.2	3.2	9	0.8	0.2	35
Papaya	14.1	2.2	11.9	0.6	0.3	56
Pomegranate	11.4	2.4	9	1	0.7	50
Pomello	9.1	1	8.1	0.7	0	36
Raspberries	7.3	4	3.3	0.7	0.4	32
Strawberries	5.8	1.5	4.3	0.5	0.2	24

Table 3: Selected Cheese

Cheese	Serving size	Carbs g	Protein g	Fat g	Energy Calories
Asaigo	1 oz.	0.9	7	11	131
Brie	1 oz.	0.1	6	8	95
Cheddar	1 oz.	0.4	7	10	115
Cottage	1 oz.	1	3	1	28
Cottage	½ cup	4	12	5	103
Feta	1 oz.	1.2	4	6	75
Gorgonzola	1 oz.	0.7	6	8	100
Gouda	1 oz.	0.6	7	8	101
Havarti	1 oz.	0.3	6	10	119
Mozzarella	1 oz.	0.7	6	7	90
Parmesan	1 oz.	0.9	10	7	111
Provolone	1 oz.	0.6	7	8	100
Queso Blanco	1 oz.	0.7	6	7	88
Ricotta	1 oz.	0.9	3	4	49
Ricotta	½ cup	4	14	16	214

7.3 Tips for Dining Out and Traveling

Eating out, socializing and traveling are parts of our life, and they all involve food. When you embark on the MRP or GRP, they can bring feelings of anxiety and stress. The tips below will help you add your new way of eating to social life without the stress or fear of standing out.

Mindset.

The first tip has to do with your mindset around the new dietary approach you are taking. It's all about how you view it, and how you present it to your friends and the people you come across. What do I mean by this? If you think or say *"I'm on this low carb diet,"* you will come across as a dieter; hence, people will not give much support or show you too much understanding. If you think about it and present it as *"I recently found out I'm severely carbohydrate intol-erant and the best way to heal my body is to eliminate carbohydrates"* (just like a gluten intolerant person would eliminate gluten), people will have an easier time understanding why you may need to abstain from certain foods. They will be less judgmental, perhaps even curious to know more about it, and will be willing to support you the best that they can.

Choose restaurants wisely.

If possible, choose places that serve vegetables and meats or seafood. Indian and Mexican restaurants are difficult to find low carb dishes. Indian foods of-ten include starches. Mexican food has few vegetables. All the other restau-rants/cuisines will usually have salads and vegetables as main dishes or sides.

Don't be afraid to ask.

You will often have to request a replacement (e.g. instead of the starch they offer, you'll ask for a vegetable or a salad). Don't be afraid to do that. It's often done; you are neither the first nor the last with such a request.

Be specific.

When you order, be specific about no sauces or have them on the side. Sauces are dangerous. They almost always contain sugar and some thickening agent that is carbohydrate-based, as well as vegetable oils. It is easier and safer to ask for grilled meats and butter or olive oil on the side.

For the salads, ask for the dressing on the side as well or, better, no dressing, just lemon/lime and olive oil, and you add them to the salad.

You can always ask them for steamed vegetables and olive oil, salt and pepper to add to the vegetables.

If you choose sautéed vegetables, ask if they can make them in butter.

Grilled vegetables are another good option.

If you want a burger, many places offer bun-less burgers. If not, just ask for it without the bun, to be served on a bed of lettuce instead.

Check out the side dishes on the menu.

Always check the side dishes. You will most likely be able to find some form of non-starchy vegetable in there. I often order 2 or 3 side vegetables when I eat out. They are less expensive than a main course.

Parties, travel, and social events.

If you go to a party that allows you to bring a dish, then take with you a plate that will have foods you can eat.

Sometimes it's a good idea to eat something at home before going to an event that you are not sure of the food they will serve.

Always keep in mind that you are there to socialize, to meet new people, or enjoy old friends, not for the sole reason of eating.

If you travel, the most important thing is to have access to good water.

Pack with you snacks like meat, cheese sticks, nuts, and seeds. On my long flights, I always travel with sardines.

7.4 Mindset & the Emotions of Change

The emotional part of adopting such lifestyle change is the biggest one. This is the first one you will need to master. Master your mind! Master your thoughts and your beliefs about your new food and lifestyle.

At first, you will feel a bit awkward. You will have the impression that all eyes are on you, but I promise you they are not.

Be strong in your beliefs. Have a clear why. Be consistent in your actions. As you keep in mind the big picture, focus on "today," focus on the "now." With time, it gets easier. You'll start to feel better. You'll grow more confident in you and your decision making. The hunger and the cravings will diminish and eventually go away. You'll feel in complete control over food, the exact opposite of what you are probably experiencing now. You will not feel deprived. Be patient and stick with it.

You may think, *"What do you know? You are a nutritionist. You've never struggled with weight, food cravings and emotional eating."* My relationship with food, was not always a healthy one. Do you think that eating a pint of ice cream the night before going for a 50-mile bike ride shows I had any control over food? Why didn't I eat only a scoop or two? Because I couldn't stop there. I wanted the whole pint. It was too good. I didn't think about any of the effects it had on my body, except for the pleasure of eating it. I wasn't worried about gaining weight, because I knew I was going to "burn it off" the next day on the bike. Yes, I had that mentality: *"exercise so you can eat."*

I really think there are very few people out there that have a perfect healthy relationship with food. I wasn't one of them, but I can say that now, after 5 years of eating nutrient dense, low carb, high fat foods, that I have the healthiest relationship with food I can ever remember. And you can, too!

Once you get your body in a fat adapted state and your brain on ketones, the magic happens. You will think you are not human anymore. *We associate being human with being tired and having guilty pleasures (at least when it comes to food).* The day you get up with energy and go to sleep with energy, you eat and don't feel guilty about it, and you have an overall feeling of peace and calm, is the day you will be saying, *"what is this, am I not human anymore?"* Let me give you a personal example so you understand what I mean by "not human."

In October 2015, I had my first "non-human experience." I enrolled in an 85-mile bike ride on behalf of the MS Foundation, part of the MS 150 ride in North Florida. It wasn't my first long distance ride. In my vegan-vegetarian years, I had done the MS 150 and I'd done a century ride. However, it was my first long distance ride done after I had my son. Not only that, but it was my first long distance ride in my new state as a "fat burning woman."

On the morning of the ride, I had a bulletproof coffee, and then I got my bike with two bottles of water and joined the roughly 2000 other people who signed up for the ride. I got on the bike at 8am and started riding, full of joy and excitement. From my training, I already expected to ride 50 miles without the need to stop for water or a restroom break. After mile 50, I became curious and interested in how the rest of the ride would go, almost like an outside observer. *When will I get tired? When will I need to stop to refuel*

How long will I be able to ride without taking a break to rest and to refresh my legs? All those questions started to pop into my mind. I became my own case study.

Is it possible for a human to ride 85 miles in a fasted state without taking any breaks?

Will I be able to do that?

I started to think that it was possible, but I had to prove it. Almost 5 hours later, I got the answer to all of my questions. Yes, it was! I finished the ride in one straight shot and in a fasted state. All I had throughout the ride was water. I had incredible physical and mental energy. A lot of it was mind over body. I believe my thoughts created my reality, although in this case my legs helped tremendously. I told myself all the time, before and during the ride: *"I can do this, it's easy and it's fun."* I tuned into what I call "the flow": the zone of unlimited potential. When I got off the bike, I felt incredibly fresh. I was "high" from such an incredible experience. I couldn't believe I'd done it! And that was the first time when I felt like I wasn't human.

At the end of previous rides, I always felt exhausted and in pain, like a bulldozer had run me over about 10 times. To finish the ride without stopping at any rest stop and not having to take any external fuel was surreal. That was my AHA moment! That's when I realized the power of food. Not only had I healed my guy and my mood, but I optimized my body's physical potential and performance.

 hope my story will inspire you to take on your own healing with foods journey vith patience, confidence, strong belief, and to be consistent in your actions.)ne day your story will inspire another person to take on their own healing ourney.

Ve are all on the same journey but at different points. For some, it brings along ealth they never dreamed of having; for others it brings a baby or more. Some get surprised with physical performance; others get to lose a lot of their body-weight.

You never know what the journey will reveal for you, but you've got to be on it to see where it takes you.

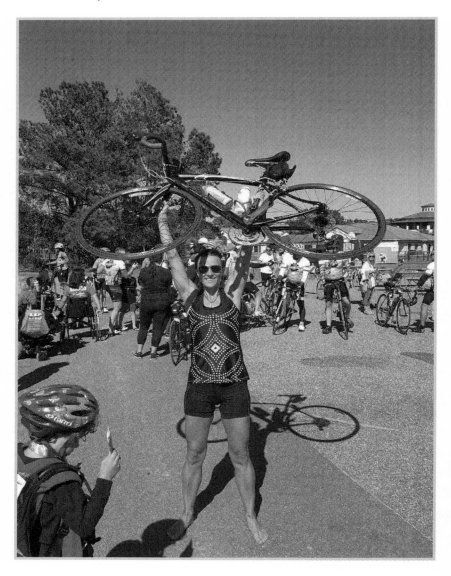

7.5 Supplements

Supplements, as the name implies, come to supplement something that is already in place. I know there is as big a push out there for supplements as there is for drugs. Many people look at supplements as a quick fix. My approach is slightly different, and by now you probably understand what that is: food and lifestyle first! With that being said, there are a few supplements that I think we all can benefit from taking on a regular basis, almost as a "security blanket."

Vitamin D3.

The best way to approach Vitamin D supplementation is to first measure your blood levels of Vitamin D (25-hydroxy Vitamin D). Based on your results, take the correct amount of Vitamin D3 to help you reach or maintain optimal levels without risking overdosing and developing toxicity. Keep in mind vitamin D is a powerful hormone; so more is not necessarily better.

The Institute for Functional Medicine has developed a sliding scale to help determine the amount of vitamin D3 needed in a supplemental form according to an individual's blood levels. I use this scale with my clients with very good results. I recommend finding a functional medicine practitioner that will be able to assist you with this.

When it comes to Vitamin D supplementation, I prefer the liquid, emulsified form, paired with its cousin, Vitamin K2.

Your best source of Vitamin D, with no risk of overdosing, is sun exposure. When you can, expose your skin (without sunscreen on) to the sun gradually early in the day and late in the evening. As you develop a suntan, then you can increase your sun exposure time and allow your body to naturally produce Vitamin D from the cholesterol in your skin.

Therapeutic strength probiotics.

You will want to take therapeutic strength probiotics along with fermented foods to assure that you inoculate your gut with healthy probiotics. Take probiotics with food. 25 billion CFU one or two times a day is a great place to start. I personally prefer the refrigerated probiotics. There are many companies out there that make probiotics. It's best to get them through a practitioner.

Fish Oil or Krill Oil.

Take these for the omega-3 anti-inflammatory fats. As maintenance, I recommend 2-3 grams a day total. That includes the DHA (about 1.2 g) and the EPA (about 1.3 g). Depending on your unique health needs (inflammation, joint, cardiovascular, or diabetes), you may take more.

Look for oils that don't have added fillers and other oil carriers, and ensure they have the breakdown of the two components: DHA & EPA.

Fermented Cod Liver Oil (FCLO).

Unlike fish oil, which is a highly-refined product, FCLO is a whole food supplement. It provides all the fat-soluble vitamins (A, D, E, K), and small amounts of omega-3. FCLO is mainly a good source of Vitamin A. It is a fermented product, which makes it more potent than a regular, refined (odorless, tasteless) cod liver oil you may find in stores.

My go-to company for FCLO is Green Pastures. They have it in liquid form, which I know most people turn their noses up to, but they also carry capsules.

Digestive enzymes.

Take these only if you need assistance digesting foods. These are on a case by case basis. You will most likely need to take digestive enzymes if you struggle with gas, bloating, diarrhea /constipation, indigestion and acid reflux. Look for a comprehensive one that has enzymes to help break down all three macronutrients, as well as cellulose, double sugars, peptides, etc.

OX bile.

This is a supplement that many of my clients go on at the beginning stages when adding more fat to their diet, especially if their gallbladder was removed. This assists with fat emulsification and digestion.

Magnesium.

It is a crucial mineral involved in hundreds of metabolic reactions in the body from energy metabolism to nerve and muscle function. You name it, magnesium is needed.

Magnesium as a supplement is sold in many forms, e.g. citrate, citramate, glycinate, etc. If constipation is one of the gut issues you struggle with Mg-citrate is the best form to help with bowel movements. If your bowel movements are well regulated, Mg-threonate is the form that's best absorbed with the least gut irritating effect.

L-carnitine.

This is a supplement you may need to take for a short period of time if you have a hard time switching over your metabolism to burning fat. If you are fatigued, have low energy, and are unable to produce ketone bodies despite following the low carb and IF plan for over 3 weeks, take this.

There are laboratory tests that measure blood levels of carnitine that you can do to assess the need for supplementation. Think of carnitine as a transporter. It takes long chain fatty acids (LCFA) from outside of the mitochondria and transports them inside where they are then used as fuel and turned into ketone bodies. The body naturally produces carnitine. Some foods like eggs and meats are a good source of the precursor amino acids (lysin and arginin). But, if your own production is not enough to help you effectively burn fats to ketones, then for a limited time, you can try to take L-carnitine at about 500-1500 mg/day.

Supplements quality

There are several supplement companies that sell their products only through healthcare practitioners. I suggest taking this healing journey with a practitioner that is well versed in what you are trying to achieve with food and lifestyle. In this case, it will be someone that has experience in implementing the MR and GR protocol(s), and they will be able to assist you in getting good quality supplements as well.

It is a jungle out there when it comes to supplements. You walk in some health food stores and they have aisles and aisles of supplements. Which one do you trust? Which one should you go with? Plus, there is no regulation on the supplement industry, so it's hard to know what they actually pack inside those tablets, capsules, soft gels, etc. If you choose to buy from a store or online, look for companies that have third party testing.

NSF, for example, is the only American National Standard that establishes requirements for the ingredients in dietary and nutritional supplements.[48]

7.6 One Week Menu

This menu fits well with the metabolic and the gut reset protocol.

When I created this menu, I had in mind a transition from a standard American diet (SAD), which provides well over 200 g of carbs a day, to a low carb diet that will keep you at around 50 g or less Net Carbs a day. This menu will allow you to ease into the low carb, whole foods.

The intention behind this 1 week menu is to:

☐ Provide you with a template for you to follow to create your own menu;

☐ Help you eat a 100% whole foods diet;

☐ Illustrate how you can use leftover dinners for the next day's lunch (cook less, eat more);

☐ Show you how to incorporate a small amount of fruit or honey into your new lifestyle;

☐ Remind you that, occasionally, you can enjoy a glass of dry wine (reserve this for when your liver is clear of fats and blood triglycerides are way below 100);

☐ Show you how you can incorporate healing foods like the chicken stock, beef soup, liver, oxtail, and fermented vegetables to your whole foods metabolic reset plan, and make it so they support gut healing.

Please feel free to make substitutions based on food availability, your personal preferences and food tolerances. I think by now you have a good understanding of the fundamental principles that make a MR or GR meal. Allow your imagination and creative cooking power to take over. *Cook with love, eat with love and heal with love.*

Meal	Day 1
Breakfast	Hemp-Berries-Greens Blast (half recipe)
Lunch	Quick Kale Salad (246 g)
	2 Hard-Boiled Eggs
Snack	¼ cup Macadamia Nuts
Dinner	Slow Cooker Oxtail (4 oz.)
	Roasted Mixed Vegetables
	with Turmeric (half recipe)
	Radish Salad (half recipe)
	¼ cup Sauerkraut Juice or Beetroot Kvass

Total Daily Intake	1790 cal	146 g fat	64 g protein	65 g carbs	25 g fiber	**40 g NC**

Meal	Day 2
Breakfast	2 Eggs Over Easy, cooked in 1 tbsp. coconut oil
	1 Hass Avocado
	¼ cup Sauerkraut
Lunch	Slow Cooker Oxtail (4 oz.)
	Mixed Greens Instant Salad (half recipe)
	Baked Beets (1 oz.)
Snack	3 tbsp. Almond Butter
Dinner	Green Beans Beef Soup (1 cup)
	Eggplant Cheesy Sandwiches (300 g or 11 oz.)
	Dino Kale Salad (half recipe)

Total Daily Intake	1670 cal	137 g fat	74 g protein	58 g carbs	28 g fiber	**30 g NC**

Meal	Day 3					
Breakfast	Arugula Pineapple Morning Blast (half recipe)					
Lunch	Cheese Eggplant Sandwich (300 g)					
Snack	1 Boiled Egg					
Dinner	Steamed Turmeric Cauliflower & Broccoli (half recipe)					
	Garlic-Dill Alaskan Baked Salmon (5 oz.)					
	Avocado Dip (half recipe)					
	Radish Salad (half recipe)					
Total Daily Intake	1900 cal	166 g fat	58 g protein	63 g carbs	25 g fiber	**38 g NC**

Meal	Day 4					
Breakfast	Cottage Cheese with Sour Cream, Honey and Cinnamon (½ recipe)					
	½ cup Organic Raspberries (to garnish)					
	2 tbsp. Hemp Seeds (to garnish)					
Lunch	Alaskan Salmon Salad (4 oz.)					
	Dino Kale Salad (full recipe)					
	Avocado Dip (4 oz.)					
Snack	¼ cup Pecans					
Dinner	Better Than Mama's Cabbage (5 oz.)					
	Baked Meatballs (4 oz.)					
	Sauerkraut (¼ cup) or Kimchi					
Total Daily Intake	1700 cal	140 g fat	62 g protein	61 g carbs	25 g fiber	36 g NC

Meal	Day 5					
Breakfast	VeggEgg Muffin (2 muffins)					
Lunch	Better Than Mama's Cabbage (5 oz.) Baked Meatballs (4 oz.) Dill Cucumber Salad (161 g) 1 Hass Avocado					
Snack	5 Brazil Nuts					
Dinner	Quick Brussel Sprouts (4 oz.) Baked Chicken Wings (3 oz.) Radish Salad (half recipe) 1 cup Homemade Chicken Stock					
Total Daily Intake	1680 cal	137 g fat	74 g protein	48 g carbs	22 g fiber	26 g NC

Meal	Day 6					
Breakfast	Zucchini Velvet Pancakes topped with Mixed Berry Sauce (about 1 oz.) Ginger Tea/Green Tea					
Lunch	Quick Brussel Sprouts (4 oz.) Baked Chicken Wings (4 oz.) Tomato Avocado Salad (full recipe)					
Snack	Sharp Cheddar Cheese (2 oz.)					
Dinner	Liver Delight (130 g) Grilled Asparagus (5 oz.) Arugula Salad (5 oz.) Red Dry Wine (e.g. Malbec - 4 oz.)					
Total Daily Intake	1750 cal	129 g fat	76 g protein	64 g carbs	26 g fiber	38 g NC

Meal	Day 7
Breakfast	Mihaela's Allspice Fat Coffee
Lunch	Sardines in Water (1 can)
	Mixed Greens Instant Salad (½ recipe)
Snack	Chicken Stock, homemade (1 cup)
Dinner	Walnut Crusted Flounder (4 oz.)
	Garlic-Lemon Sauce (2 tbsp.)
	Sautéed Spinach with Garlic (half recipe)
	Chia Seeds Pudding
Total daily intake	1632 cal · 138 g fat · 63 g protein · 53 g carbs · 30 g fiber · 23 g NC

Note: On a day like day 7, when you begin to add intermittent fasting and are able to bring your NC to less than 30 g, and you may not get enough fiber, you can add 3 tbsp. of chia seeds for additional fiber. You can simply mix it in water, or have the chia pudding.

7.7 Recipes

Shakes, Eggs and More

Tips for green blasts/shakes/smoothies

As a general rule use 50% greens, 15% fruits, 35% nuts/seeds/butters/oils, and water to reach the desired consistency (1-2 cups). If you prefer a thick consistency, so you can eat it with a spoon, use less or no water. If you like a thin consistency, so you can drink it through a straw, add more water.

For extra flavor, you can add cinnamon, ginger, nutmeg, cayenne pepper, turmeric, chlorella, cacao, etc. You can also add olive oil, coconut oil, cacao butter, flax oil or hemp oil. The nuts and oils will slow down the absorption of the sugar from the fruits, and the insulin response to it will be milder. It will also make you feel full for a longer time and you'll get all of the oil's wonderful health benefits, too! Use ingredients you have available and play with it. Just remember to follow the 50%, 15%, 35% rule. You will be surprised at the tasty combinations you'll come up with!

Hemp Berry Greens Blast

Makes 2 servings / Net Carbs per serving: 22 g

Ingredients:

1 handful of mixed greens of your choice

1 small ripe banana — *more ?*

1 cup mixed frozen organic berries

1 slice beet root (1 inch thick)

Juice from ½ Maier lemon

1 scoop Deeper Greens [*whole foods based antioxidant powder (optional)]

3 tbsp. hemp seeds

1 cup Water — *less*

*You can use chlorella or spirulina

Directions:

Place all the ingredients in the large *Nutribullet container.

Add coconut water to MAX line.

Blend for maximum 1 minute.

Serve immediately.

If you don't have a Nutribullet, use a regular blender, and just add water to each desired consistency.

Arugula Pineapple Blast

Makes 2 servings / Net Carbs per serving: 15 g

Ingredients:

> 1 cup packed baby arugula
>
> ½ cup chopped pineapple
>
> ¼ cup pine nuts
>
> 1 pinch Celtic sea salt
>
> 1 cup water
>
> 1 date
>
> Use green stevia if you want a non-caloric sweetener.

Directions:

Place all the ingredients in the Vita-Mix (or any blender you have).

Add water to reach desired consistency.

Blend and serve immediately. You can use ice if you want a cold beverage.

Cottage Cheese with Sour Cream, Honey & Cinnamon

Makes 2 servings / Net Carbs: 11 g

Ingredients:

> ½ cup cottage cheese (from organic, grass-fed cows)
>
> 1 tbsp. sour cream (from organic, grass-fed cows)
>
> ½ tbsp. medicinal honey (raw)

¼ tsp. vanilla extract

½ tsp. cinnamon

2-3 drops of essential oil (optional: Citrus Fresh by Young Living)

Directions:

Place all the ingredients in a glass bowl, mix well and serve.

Garnish with fresh organic raspberries and hemp seeds.

Eggs Over Easy with Avocado, Tomato and Sauerkraut

Makes 1 Serving / Net Carbs: 8 g

Ingredients:

2 eggs

1 Hass avocado

1 medium tomato

¼ cup sauerkraut

1 tbsp. coconut oil (or grass fed butter or ghee)

Salt and pepper to taste

Cayenne pepper (optional)

Directions:

Heat the coconut oil in a frying pan (preferably stainless steel, ceramic or cast iron).

Place the eggs in the pan.

Add salt, pepper, and cayenne.

When the egg white is all cooked on the side facing up, flip the eggs with a spatula onto the other side and cook for few more seconds—just enough to cook the remaining egg white.

Turn the heat off and serve immediately with slices of avocado, tomato and sauerkraut.

VeggEgg Muffin

Makes 6 servings / Net Carbs per serving 2 g

One serving = 1 muffin

Ingredients:

> 6 eggs
>
> 3 green onions, minced
>
> ½ cup bell peppers, diced small
>
> 1 tbsp. of fat of your choice, (butter, coconut oil, ghee, etc.)
>
> 1/2 cup lightly steamed and chopped broccoli (or any other vegetable you have available and you like)
>
> Cilantro minced (or any herb you like)
>
> ½ tsp. salt (or less)
>
> ¼ tsp. ground black pepper
>
> 1 tsp. turmeric
>
> ¼ cup grated cheese of your choice

Directions:

Preheat oven to 350°F (175°C).

Line a muffin tin with non-bleached paper or silicone liners.

In a skillet over medium heat, soften the onions in the fat for about 5 minutes.

When they are translucent, add the bell peppers, and cook on medium heat until they begin to soften.

Remove from the heat.

Mix the eggs with salt, pepper and turmeric and whisk with a fork until well combined. Optional use a blender.

Now it's time to build the muffins: fill up each muffin cup with a spoonful of onion/bell pepper/broccoli/cilantro/cheese. Evenly distribute the filling to 6 muffin cups.

Pour the egg mixture into each cup until about ¾ of the cup is full.

Bake for about 30 minutes or until fully set.

The cups will come out puffed up and then fall a bit as they cool.

Kale and Cheese Casserole

Makes 4 servings / Net Carbs per serving: 8 g

serving = 337 g

Ingredients:

8 eggs, beaten

¼ cup butter

1 pound fresh kale, washed and chopped

¾ cup whole milk cheddar cheese, shredded (organic and grass fed if available)

½ cup heavy cream (organic and grass fed if available)

1 tbsp. chopped fresh basil (or ½ tsp. dried basil)

¾ cup chopped cherry tomatoes

¾ cup shredded whole milk mozzarella (organic and grass fed, if available)

¼ cup thinly sliced scallions

¼ tsp. salt

¼ tsp. pepper

Directions:

Preheat oven to 350° F.

Melt butter in large skillet.

Add kale, salt and pepper.

Cook kale until wilted. Set aside.

In a large mixing bowl, combine the eggs and cheddar.

Stir in cream and basil.

Fold in the kale, tomato, mozzarella and scallions.

Spread evenly in a greased baking dish (2-quart casserole or baking dish).

Bake for 30–35 minutes or until a fork inserted near the center comes out clear

Allow to stand for 10–15 minutes before serving.

Note: You can replace kale with any greens you like. For a dairy-free version, omit the cheese. Instead of butter, use coconut oil and use coconut cream as a substitute for the heavy cream.

Zucchini Velvet Pancakes

Makes 10 pancakes / Net Carbs per serving: 4 g if made with nut milk / 3 g if made with water

Ingredients:

> 4 eggs
>
> 1 medium zucchini, steamed and pureed
>
> 3 cups walnut flour
>
> 3 tbsp. coconut oil
>
> 1 tbsp. organic beet powder
>
> ½ tsp. vanilla extract
>
> ½ tsp. baking soda
>
> Lemon juice from ½ lemon
>
> One pinch of Himalayan salt
>
> ½ cup water or ½ cup nut pine nut-hemp milk (see recipe in the Desserts section)

Directions:

Place all ingredients except for baking soda and lemon juice in a food processor.

Blend well.

Add baking soda and lemon juice, allow for the acid base reaction to take place, then mix it in the pancake batter.

In a small sauce pan, melt the coconut oil if it is solid.

Cook pancakes until bubbles form on top, then flip and cook for another minute or so.

Top the pancakes with mixed berry sauce (recipe below).

Mixed Berry Sauce

Serving size: 1 oz. / Net Carbs per serving: 5 g

Ingredients:

> 1 cup of fresh or frozen raspberries
>
> 1 tbsp. of honey

Directions:

Place berries and honey in a blender.

Add water to reach a sauce like consistency.

Mihaela's Allspice Fat Coffee

Makes 1 serving /NC per serving 0 g

Ingredients:

> 8 oz. freshly made coffee using the Italian mocha French press or espresso machine
>
> 1 tbsp. grass-fed butter
>
> 1 tbsp. coconut oil (preferably virgin unrefined organic)

1/4 tsp. allspice or pumpkin spice

Stevia to sweeten (optional)

*I drink mine without any sweetener!

Directions:

Blend all the ingredients together for 30 seconds using a bullet or a blender.

Soups and Salads.

Chicken Stock/Broth

Makes 4 quarts / 1 cup serving has 0.9 g NC

Ingredients:

1 whole chicken

6 chicken feet (optional, but highly recommended)

1 whole onion

3 large carrots

4-6 small *parsley roots

1 medium *celery root (celeriac)

^Salt to taste

1 tsp. Peppercorns

*if you are unable to find parsley and celery roots, you can still make the stock. Other things you can add to it to increase flavor and add to its healing power are: kombu, shitake mushrooms, ginger and turmeric root.

^When I make a stock, I use an 8 quart soup pot; I fill it up with water to the handles and for that amount of stock I use 1 heaping tbsp. of Himalayan or Celtic salt.

Directions:

Cut the chicken legs and wings off the carcass. Put the carcass inside the soup pot.

Cut the nails off the feet.

Place chicken feet in an 8-quart soup pot together with the carcass (neck and back). I recommend using a stainless steel pot.

Add water to fill up the pot, leaving about 2 inches room on the top.

Bring it to a boil.

Skim off the foam that forms when it begins to boil.

After you skim it, add the salt and the peppercorns to the boiling mixture. Cover with a lid and simmer for 3 hours.

Peel all the vegetables, but do not chop them.

After 3-4 hours of simmering the chicken and the chicken feet, add the vegetables to the chicken base.

Bring it back to a boil, then cover with the lid and continue to simmer for 1½-2 hours max.

Turn the heat off.

Let the soup cool off a little, then strain it through a dense sieve.

Use the broth as a drink/the best gut and immune system medicine, or as base for vegetable soups and other dishes.

Note: For extra flavor, you can use the greens from the parsley and celery root, tie them with a cotton string and add them to the soup in the last half hour of cooking. Discard them at the end.

To make beef stock or any other stock, use the same recipe; just adjust the cooking time, with less time for smaller and younger animals, and longer time for larger and older animals. As an example, you will boil the large beef bones for 8-12 hours before adding the vegetables.

Green Bean Beef Soup

Makes 12 servings / Net carbs per serving: 4 g

One serving = 1 cup or 250 g

Ingredients:

2 quarts of beef broth (homemade)

1 lb. green beans

2 medium carrots

1 red bell pepper

1 medium onion

2 celery stalks

2 large tomatoes, chopped

4-5 cloves of garlic, minced

Salt and pepper to taste

Directions:

Peel, clean, and chop all vegetables into bite size pieces.

In a skillet, add a small amount of the fat that accumulates on top of the broth when it's cold. Sauté all the vegetables, except for tomatoes, garlic and parsley, until they get soft and translucent.

Place the broth in a soup pot, bring it to a boil, and add the sautéed vegetables to it. Then reduce heat and simmer for 10-15 minutes.

Add chopped tomatoes. Cook for another 5 minutes.

Add garlic and parsley.

Turn the heat off and let it cool.

Serve with sour cream or yogurt.

You can use fresh parsley, cilantro, or any fresh herb you like to garnish.

Note: Add salt and pepper only as needed. You can also add to this soup sauerkraut instead of sour cream. You may substitute the beef broth with chicken or any broth you prefer.

Arugula Salad

Makes 2 servings / Net Carbs per serving: 8 g

Ingredients:

> 1 head of romaine lettuce
>
> 4 oz. of arugula (you don't need to measure this, just use as much as you like)
>
> 1 small roasted beetroot
>
> ¼ cup walnuts
>
> Apple cider vinegar or lemon juice
>
> Truffle oil

Salt and pepper to taste

Shaved parmesan or gorgonzola cheese (optional)

Directions:

Chop the romaine lettuce into 1 inch chunks.

Place it in a large salad bowl and add the arugula.

Cut the beetroot into small cubes and add it to the salad bowl.

Add the walnuts.

In a small jar, mix the vinegar/lemon juice and truffle oil with the salt and pepper, then pour over the salad and toss well.

Sprinkle with shaved parmesan cheese or add gorgonzola cheese (optional).

Dino Kale Salad

Makes 2 servings / Net Carbs per serving: 9 g

Ingredients:

1 bunch of kale, sliced (Lacinato, "dinosaur," cavolo nero) mid-ribs removed

2/3 cup grated Pecorino Romano cheese or other flavorful grating cheese, such as Manchego or Parmesan

Juice of 1 lemon

¼ cup extra-virgin olive oil

2 cloves garlic, minced

Salt and pepper to taste

Hot red pepper flakes to taste

Directions:

Whisk together lemon juice, olive oil, garlic, salt, pepper and a generous pinch of hot red pepper flakes.

Pour over kale in serving bowl and massage the kale until it gets softer.

Add the cheese and toss again.

Let kale sit for at least 5 minutes.

Note: For a dairy free version, omit the cheese and use nuts or seeds instead. Pine nuts and or hemp seeds are great with this type of kale. Add them at the end, after you are done massaging the kale.

Quick Kale Salad

Makes 4 servings / Net Carbs per serving: 9 g

One serving = 246 g

Ingredients:

1 bundle of organic curly kale

1 small onion

1 medium tomato

1 avocado

¼ cup walnut pieces

1 tbsp. Dulse flakes

¼ cup olive oil (first cold-pressed extra virgin)

Juice from 1 lemon

Salt and pepper to taste

Directions:

Wash kale, remove the stems, and chop or slice into bite size pieces.

In a separate container, whisk together lemon juice, olive oil, salt, pepper and dulse flakes.

In a large bowl, massage the kale with the dressing until kale gets nice and soft.

Chop the onion and tomato, then add to the massaged kale. Cut avocado in big chunks and add to salad. Add the walnuts and toss well.

Let it sit for about 5-10 minutes before eating.

Note: You may add boiled eggs to the salad or eat them on the side if you choose to cook them soft. A higher fat variation would be to add 2 tbsp. mayonnaise to the hard-boiled eggs and make an egg salad.

Radish Salad

Makes 2 servings / Net Carbs per serving: 2 g

Ingredients:

2-3 bunches of radishes

¼ cup olive oil

Juice from 1 lemon

Salt and pepper to taste

Directions:

Cut the greens and trim the tips of the radishes. Rinse with cold water. Cut radishes in thin slices and place them in a glass bowl.

Add salt, pepper, and the lemon juice to the radishes and massage them well, until they get soft and juicy.

Allow it to marinate for 10-15 min, then add the olive oil, mix well.

Serve immediately or keep it in the refrigerator for later use.

Note: This salad is better the next day. The radishes become softer and release more of their spicy sulfur containing compounds.

Tomato and Avocado Salad

Makes 2 servings / Net Carbs per serving: 3 g

Ingredients:

1 Hass avocado

1 large tomato

Olive oil

Salt and pepper to taste

Directions:

Cut avocado lengthwise into ½ inch slices. Cut tomato in half and then cut lengthwise in ½ inch slices.

Place tomato and avocado in a bowl. Add salt, pepper, and drizzle with olive oil.

Serve Immediately or chill in an airtight container before serving.

Dill Cucumber Salad

Makes 3 servings / Net Carbs per serving: 4 g

One serving = 161 g or 5.7 oz.

Ingredients:

2 medium sized cucumbers (not waxed)

1 clove of garlic

One bunch fresh dill

Salt and pepper to taste

2 tbsp. olive oil

Apple cider vinegar to taste

Directions:

Wash and clean cucumbers (peeling is optional; I like keeping the skin on).

Chop the cucumbers into small square chunks.

Chop the dill and the garlic.

In a bowl, mix the cucumbers with salt, pepper, dill, and garlic. Massage them to allow the juice to come out and the cucumbers to get soft.

Add apple cider vinegar to taste and the olive oil.

Allow it to marinate for 10-15 min.

Note: This salad gets better as it marinates and the flavors blend in.

Mixed Greens Instant Salad

Makes 2 servings / Net Carbs per serving: 8 g

Ingredients:

½ pound mixed baby greens

3 green onions or ¼ small red onion

1 avocado

1 tomato

Juice from 1 lemon

4 tbsp. olive oil

Salt and pepper to taste

Directions:

Place the greens in a large bowl.

Chop the tomato, avocado and onion, add them to the bowl with the greens.

Add the lemon juice, salt, pepper, and olive oil.

Toss lightly and serve immediately.

Note: For variations of this, you can use garlic instead of onion and add fresh herbs like dill, parsley or cilantro. For additional protein and fat, you can always add walnuts or hemp seeds, olives and gorgonzola cheese. For a sweet flavor add a small amount of baked beets.

Main Dishes

Garlic Dill Wild Alaskan Salmon

Makes 3 servings /Net Carbs per serving: 1 g

Ingredients:

1 lb. Wild Caught Alaskan Salmon

4 oz. of Garlic-Dill Butter (see recipe in Sauces and Dips section)

1 lemon, cut into slices (enough to garnish the plate)

Celtic sea salt/Himalayan crystal salt and pepper to taste

1-2 tbsp. of organic coconut oil or grass fed butter

Fresh dill to garnish the plate

174 g Avocado Dip (see recipe on page 349)

Directions:

Preheat the oven to 350°F.

Cover the bottom of a ceramic or glass baking dish with a thin layer of butter or coconut oil. Sprinkle with some salt and pepper. Place the salmon skin side down in the dish. Cover the fish with slices of Garlic-Dill Butter. Bake for 10-15 minutes depending on the thickness.

Take the salmon out of the oven just before it is fully cooked, as it will continue to cook after you take it out.

Allow it to slightly cool and then spread some of the avocado dip over the salmon.

Garnish with fresh dill and sliced lemon.

Wild Alaskan Salmon Salad

Makes 1 serving / Net carbs per serving: 1 g

Ingredients:

4 oz. Wild Alaskan Salmon

4 tbsp. mayonnaise (see recipe in the Sauces and Dips section)

Directions:

In a bowl, mix the salmon with the mayonnaise, and use a fork to mash it.

Add more spices if needed.

Serve over a bed of leafy salad greens or the Dino Kale Salad.

Note: For this salad, you can use leftover salmon or, if you don't have any leftovers, you can use a small can of wild Alaskan salmon. Try to buy one that comes in a BPA free can. If you plan to buy mayonnaise from the store, I recommend The Primal Kitchen brand.

Walnut Crusted Flounder

Makes 4 servings / Net Carbs per serving 0.7 g

One serving = 4.6 oz.

Ingredients:

1 lb. Flounder filet

½ cup walnut flour

Salt and pepper to taste

1-2 tbsp. garlic-lemon sauce (see recipe in Sauces and Dips section)

Directions:

Preheat the oven to 350°F.

Mix the salt and pepper with the walnut flour.

Coat the flounder well on both sides with the mixture.

Place the fish in a baking dish with parchment paper and bake at 350°F for 15 minutes.

Allow it to breathe outside of the oven for 5 minutes, and then serve.

Top with garlic-lemon sauce before serving.

Slow Cooker Oxtail

Makes 8 servings / Net Carbs per serving: 0.5 g

One serving is 171 g or 6 oz.

Ingredients:

>   3 lbs. oxtail cut (from grass fed pasture raised beef – most places sell it pre-cut)

>   4 cloves of garlic, minced

>   Salt and pepper to taste

>   Hungarian paprika

>   Water, just enough to cover half the height of the solid ingredients

Directions:

Wash the oxtail in cold water, drain it, and place it in the slow cooker. Add the spices and garlic (chopped or pressed through a garlic press).

Cover ½ to ¾ with water and cook on the low setting for 7 hours.

Baked Meatballs

Makes 6 servings / Net Carbs per serving: 1 g

One serving = 3 meatballs or about 177 g

Ingredients:

> 2 pounds ground meat (50/50 beef and pork) or pan sausages
>
> 2 eggs
>
> Salt and pepper to taste (if you use pan sausages, you don't need to add any salt or pepper)
>
> 2 cloves garlic, minced (optional)
>
> A small bunch of fresh parsley, finely chopped

Directions:

Preheat the oven to 350°F.

Line a baking tray with parchment paper.

In a large bowl, mix the ground meat with the eggs and all the spices.

Form the mixture into balls and place them in the tray. You will have approximately 18 balls. If you prefer them smaller, you can go as high as 24 balls.

Bake for about 30 minutes or until cooked through.

Baked Chicken Wings

Makes 4 servings / Net Carbs per serving: 0 g

One serving = 3 wings

Ingredients:

12 chicken wings

Salt and pepper to taste

Hungarian paprika

Turmeric powder

Garlic (optional)

Hot pepper flakes (optional)

Directions:

Preheat the oven to 350°F.

Place the wings in a roasting pan in a single layer.

In a small bowl, mix all the dry ingredients and use them to season the wings.

Cover the pan with a lid and bake for 30-40 min, or until wings are golden brown.

Note: You don't need to add extra fat or water to the pan. You may use chicken legs instead of wings.

Liver Delight

Makes 4 servings / Net Carbs per serving: 3.5 g

One serving = 130 g or 4.6 oz.

Ingredients:

1 medium onion (red, white or yellow) or 1 leek

1 small bell pepper

2 cups chicken liver

3 tbsp. butter/ghee/coconut oil

Salt and pepper to taste

Fresh dill/parsley/basil to garnish

Directions:

Soak the liver in water with lemon juice, or in homemade yogurt or whey, for a few hours, to remove the bitter taste.

Wash and dry the liver. Cut it in small pieces using scissors.

Chop the onion and the bell pepper.

In a frying pan, melt the butter/ghee/coconut oil and add the onion and the bell pepper. Cook the onion and the bell pepper until they start to turn golden and soft.

Add the liver, salt and pepper and cook for an additional 4-5 minutes.

Garnish with fresh herbs of your choice. Drizzle with olive oil (optional).

Serve immediately.

Note: If you have leftovers, you can put the liver in a food processor and blend it with olive oil to make liver pate.

Side Dishes

Grilled Asparagus

Makes 4 servings / Net Carbs per serving: 2 g

One Serving = 120 g or 4 oz.

Ingredients:

> 1 lb. asparagus
>
> 2 tbsp. butter/ghee/coconut oil
>
> Salt and pepper to taste
>
> Garlic-oil (optional)

Directions:

Preheat the oven to 350°F.

Clean the asparagus. Break off the fibrous part and place it in a baking tray.

Melt butter/ghee/coconut oil and brush the asparagus with it.

Bake at 350°F for 15 min or until cooked.

Add salt and pepper to taste.

Sprinkle with garlic-olive oil (optional).

Serve immediately. Any leftovers are great added to a salad the next day.

Note: You can garnish it with grated parmesan. If you have leftovers, they can go into any salad.

Grilled Zucchini and Yellow Summer Squash

Makes 2 servings / Net Carbs per serving: 4 g

One serving = 196 g or 7 oz.

Ingredients:

> 1 medium zucchini
>
> 1 medium yellow summer squash
>
> Salt and pepper to taste
>
> Rosemary
>
> Garlic lemon sauce

Directions:

Wash and cut lengthwise the zucchini and the summer squash. For a juicier feel, leave the slices thicker. For a more dry feel, make them thinner.

Place them on a grill and turn them to uniformly cook on both sides. If you don't have a grill, you can bake them on a baking tray covered with parchment paper at 350°F for 15-20 min or until cooked.

Sprinkle with salt, pepper and rosemary to taste.

Serve them with the garlic-lemon sauce (see recipe in the sauces section).

Roasted Mixed Vegetables

Makes 6 servings / Net Carbs per serving 2 g

One serving = ¾ cup or about 88 g

Ingredients:

> 2 lbs. seasonal non-starchy vegetables (broccoli, cauliflower, summer squash, mushrooms, eggplant etc.)
>
> ⅓ cup coconut oil
>
> ½ tsp. sea salt
>
> ½ tsp. black pepper
>
> 1 tsp. turmeric
>
> ⅓ cup chopped fresh herbs

Directions:

Preheat the oven to 350°F.

Chop vegetables so that all pieces are approximately the same size. This will ensure all vegetables finish cooking at the same time.

Melt the coconut oil and pour over the vegetables.

Toss together all ingredients and spread them in a single layer on a large roasting pan or cookie sheet.

Stirring occasionally, roast the vegetables for 40–45 minutes, or until cooked through and browned.

Note: By the strictest definition of roasting, these vegetables are blackened. To reduce the browning of foods, I choose to not cook above 350° F.

Baked Beets

Makes 7 servings / Net Carbs per serving: 2 g

One serving = 1 oz.

Ingredients:

> 4 medium sized beetroots

Directions:

Preheat the oven at 325°F for a convection oven or 350°F for a regular oven.

Clean the beetroots, and cut the top and bottom off.

Place them on a baking tray with parchment paper.

Bake them until soft all the way through.

When fully cooked, take them out and allow to cool for 5 minutes.

Peel the skin, cut in slices.

Note: Sprinkle ground cumin on top for some extra flavor. They last well in the refrigerator for 2-3 days. You can add them to any salad, soup or shake for a sweet flavor and a pinkish color.

When you are in a hurry, you can also steam the beets, as it takes less time. They will be less yummy, but still good.

Although beets are high in sugar, I recommend having them periodically in small amounts, as they are powerful detoxifiers.

Steamed Turmeric Cauliflower & Broccoli

Makes 2 servings / Net Carbs per serving: 4 g

One serving = 130 g or 4.4 oz.

Ingredients:

> 1 cup chopped broccoli
>
> 1 cup chopped cauliflower
>
> 4 tbsp. olive oil
>
> Salt and pepper to taste
>
> ½ tsp. turmeric

Directions:

Cut the broccoli and the cauliflower into florets.

Place them in the steamer and steam them for 5 min.

Remove from the steamer and place in a large mixing bowl.

Add olive oil, salt, pepper and turmeric.

Toss all the ingredients together and serve while hot.

Note: For a variation of this dish, after you steam the vegetables you can braise them in butter or coconut oil. Or you can place them in a baking dish, add butter and top with cheese and bake until the cheese melts.

Quick Brussel Sprouts

Makes 4 servings / Net Carbs per serving: 6 g

One serving = 126 g

Ingredients:

> 1 lb. brussel sprouts
>
> 3-4 tbsp. butter/ghee/coconut oil/or any animal fat left from roasting
>
> Salt and pepper to taste
>
> 1 tsp. turmeric

Directions:

Clean and cut the brussel sprouts in half or quarters. They cook faster and taste better if cut to a smaller size.

Place in a steamer and steam at low heat for 5-7 minutes, or until desired softness is reached.

Preheat the oven to 350°F.

Remove sprouts from the steamer and place on a baking dish. Add salt, pepper, turmeric, and butter/ghee.

Bake for 15 minutes, then leave it in the turned off oven for another 5-10 minutes or until you are ready to serve them.

Tip: To increase the health benefits of the Brussel sprouts, let them sit for at least 5 minutes after you cut them before steaming them.

Variation: If you wish to make this a super-fast dish, skip the baking. Just add 3-4 tbsp. of olive oil. The spices mix well right after you remove the vegetable from the steamer. Serve while hot.

Better than Mama's Cabbage

Makes 12 servings / Net Carbs per serving 7 g

One serving = 140 g or 5 oz.

Ingredients:

> 1 red small cabbage, approximately 5" diameter

> 1 white small cabbage, approximately 5" diameter

> 3 tbsp. coconut oil or butter (preferably grass fed and organic)

> Celtic sea salt and pepper to taste

Directions:

Shred the cabbage.

In a large stainless steel pan, place the oil and the cabbage. Start cooking at low heat until cabbage is soft and sweet. Do not add any water and do not cook under a cover. You will need to stir it frequently, so it doesn't burn the bottom of the pan. This will take over 30 min, so be patient and stir frequently. Add the salt and pepper halfway.

Serve immediately and store the rest in the refrigerator.

Note: It makes wonderful leftovers. This is the type of dish you cook once and eat 2 or 3 times. It gets better every time you reheat it.

never use a microwave. I reheat it in the oven or in a sauce pan on top of the stove. Because it takes a long time to make it, I like to make a lot so I have some for a few days. If you don't like eating left overs, just make ½ or ¼ of the recipe.

This cabbage is absolutely delicious; my husband says it tastes like pasta. Enjoy!

Sautéed Spinach with Garlic

Makes 2 servings / Net Carbs per serving: 4 g

One serving = 1 cup cooked

Ingredients:

2 cups steamed and chopped spinach

3 garlic cloves, sliced and crushed

3 tbsp. coconut oil

Salt and pepper to taste

Hot red pepper flakes (optional)

Directions:

In a frying pan, melt the coconut oil.

Add the garlic when the oil is hot.

Cook the garlic until it starts to turn golden.

Add the spinach, salt and pepper.

Cook for 2-3 more minutes.

Serve warm.

Note: I like to steam the spinach prior to sautéing it. It makes it easier to measure and it allows me to use a smaller frying/sauté pan.

Eggplant Cheesy Sandwiches

Makes 8 servings / Net Carbs per serving: 10 g

One serving = 300 g or 11 oz.

Ingredients:

> 2 medium eggplants
>
> 4-6 eggs
>
> 4-6 tbsp. of melted coconut oil
>
> Water, as needed
>
> 1-2 cups of walnut flour
>
> Salt and pepper to taste
>
> 8 or more tbsp. of Basic onion-tomato-basil sauce (see recipe below)
>
> 1 lb. Havarti cheese slices

Pre-directions note: This is a three step recipe. I promise it's worth taking the time to make it. The sandwiches store well in the refrigerator, and they can be easily reheated in a pan or in the oven. They are great even cold.

Step 1: Make the "breaded" eggplant

This part has three distinct steps.

- Prep the eggplant
- Make the walnut-egg mix for "breading"
- Make the "breaded" eggplant

Eggplant prep:

Cut the eggplant into ½ inch thick medallions.

Cover a baking tray with paper towels and place the eggplant on the tray.

Sprinkle with salt, and layer them with paper towels.

Allow it to sit for a minimum of 1 hour (or overnight). The salt will pull out excess liquid from the eggplant.

Drain the liquid. Now the eggplant is ready to work with.

As you're waiting for the eggplant to sit, prepare the egg and walnut mix for "breading".

Preheat the oven to 325°F for a convection oven or 350°F for a regular oven.

Prepare a baking tray with parchment paper and grease it with 2-3 tbsp. of melted coconut oil.

Walnut-egg mix

Whisk the eggs with 2-3 tbsp. of water.

Add salt and pepper to taste (remember, the eggplants are already salted from the water pulling process).

Place the walnut flour in a bowl.

The "breaded" eggplant

Dip the eggplant in egg wash, then in walnut flour, coating both sides evenly.

Place them in a single layer in the baking tray.

Drizzle with melted coconut oil.

Bake for 15-20 min or until golden brown, flipping them midway.

Allow them to cool for 5 minutes, then create the "sandwiches."

While you are baking the "breaded" eggplant, procede to prepare the basic onion-tomato-basil sauce.

Step 2: Make the basic onion-tomato-basil sauce [BOTBS]

Makes 55 servings / Net Carbs per serving: 1 g

One serving = 1 tbsp.

Ingredients:

> 3 large onions
>
> 1 red bell pepper (optional)
>
> 1 large tomato
>
> 2 tbsp. of coconut oil, grass fed butter, or ghee
>
> Fresh or dry basil to taste
>
> Salt and pepper to taste

Directions:

Chop the onion, pepper, and the tomato and set aside.

Heat a sauté pan and melt the fat of your choice (coconut oil, grass fed butter, or ghee).

Add the onion and cook at low heat covered for 15-20 min, until the onion is soft and sweet.

Add the bell pepper after about 10 min and cook together with the onion.

Add the tomato and cook uncovered for another 10 min, until all ingredients are soft and the juice is reduced.

Chop the basil and add it to the sauce.

Cover for 3 min and take it off the heat.

Allow it to cool and use it for the Eggplant Sandwiches.

Note: I use this sauce as a base for many other dishes. I add it to vegetables like mushrooms, zucchini noodles, and spaghetti squash, as well as when I make the quick liver.

Part 3: Make the Sandwiches

Cover one slice of "breaded" eggplant with about 1 tbsp. BOTBS (use more if a really big slice) and one slice of cheese. Then cover with another eggplant and create a Cheesy Eggplant "sandwich."

Repeat, until you use all sliced and "breaded" eggplants to create sandwiches.

Place the sandwiches on a baking tray covered with parchment paper and bake for 10-15 minutes, or until the cheese is melted and golden brown.

Note: You can always make open face sandwiches if you'd like.

Sauces and Dips

Avocado Dip

Makes 2 servings / Net Carbs per serving: 6 g

One serving = 174 g

Ingredients:

2 ripe avocados (Hass or California style)

2 garlic cloves, minced

¼ small onion, finely chopped

2-3 tbsp. cilantro finely chopped

Juice from 1 lemon

Salt and pepper to taste

Directions:

Peel and cut avocado in small pieces.

Place it in a bowl.

Add garlic, onion, cilantro, salt pepper and lemon juice.

Use a fork and mash all the ingredients together.

Serve fresh.

Note: If you have leftovers, to reduce browning caused by oxidation, place the dip in a small container and add the avocado pits to it. Cover and store in the refrigerator for 14 hours max.

Garlic-Dill Butter Spread

Makes 4 servings / Net Carbs per serving: 1 g

Ingredients:

4 oz. or 100 g unsalted grass fed organic butter

2-3 cloves of garlic, minced

4 tbsp. dill, finely chopped

Salt and pepper to taste

Directions:

Place butter in a bowl and allow it to soften to room temperature (about 10-15 minutes).

Chop the dill and the garlic.

In a bowl, mix the salt, pepper, dill, and garlic. Incorporate it into the butter to obtain a paste. Place the paste on a wax paper and shape it into a roll.

Place the roll in the freezer for 30 minutes or longer.

Transfer to the refrigerator 30 minutes prior to cooking with it.

Slice the roll and place over your dish (salmon, etc.).

Note: If you wish, you can make the Garlic-Dill Butter and use it right away. Just skip the freezer step.

If you have leftovers, store them in the freezer.

Garlic-Lemon Sauce:

Makes 7.4 servings / Net Carbs per serving: 0.8 g

One serving = 1 tbsp.

Ingredients:

      Juice from 1 lemon

      2-3 garlic cloves

      ¼ cup olive oil

Directions:

In a small bowl, mix pressed garlic with salt, lemon juice and olive oil.

You can use a mortar and pestle to first crush the garlic with salt and pepper, and slowly add the lemon juice to it.

After it is well crushed, slowly add the olive oil.

You may add a small amount of water if it is too thick or too strong according to your taste. Whisk well, until it turns milky white.

Pour the sauce over your desired dish before serving.

Mayonnaise

Makes 7 servings / Net Carbs per serving: 0.4 g

One serving = 2 tbsp.

Ingredients:

      2 egg yolks

      ¾ cups olive oil

¼ tsp. salt

Pinch of pepper

2-3 tsp. mustard

½ tsp. lemon juice

Directions:

Separate the egg yolk from the whites.

Mix the egg yolk with olive oil in a food processor or by hand.

Add the oil very slowly and allow it to be incorporated by the yolk.

Add salt, lemon juice and mustard to taste.

Mix well until all the ingredients are well incorporated.

Use immediately and store the remaining in a glass jar with an airtight lid.

Note: If the mayonnaise "breaks," add 2-3 cubes of ice to it and continue to blend it.

Ferments

Sauerkraut

Ingredients:

> 1 organic white cabbage
>
> 1 organic red cabbage
>
> Salt to taste (about 1 tsp. for 1½ cabbages, preferably Celtic sea salt or Himalayan crystal salt)
>
> Thyme and dill, preferably fresh
>
> Horseradish (2 inch long root)
>
> 1-2 quart glass jar

Directions:

Shred the cabbage with a knife or in a food processor. Peel and slice the horse-radish length wise, in ½ inch slices. They will look like tick sticks.

In a large bowl, knead the cabbage with the salt well with your hands until a lot of cabbage juice is expressed.

On the bottom of a jar, lay thyme and fresh dill.

Add the slices of horseradish (peeled).

Pack the cabbage mixture into the glass jar, leaving about 1½-2 inches at the top empty, as the cabbage will expand with fermentation.

Press firmly so there is no air trapped and the cabbage is drowned into its own juice.

If there is not enough juice to cover the cabbage, add some salty water (brine).

You can add more slices of horseradish to the sides of the jar. This will give a certain spice and will prevent the cabbage from getting soft and slimy.

Close the jar with a lid—not too tight to allow the fermentation gases to escape.

Cover the jar with a kitchen towel to create a dark environment.

Keep it at room temperature to allow it to ferment. Best fermentation takes place at around 74-78°F.

Note: It will take 7-10 days for the sauerkraut to be ready on the kitchen counter, at room temperature, covered with a towel.

Enjoy it with meats and eggs. You can add it to the soups and salads as well.

Sauerkraut Juice

Ingredients:

> Organic white and red cabbage
>
> Salt to taste (Celtic sea salt or Himalayan crystal salt)
>
> Fresh thyme and dill preferably, if not available dry is ok too
>
> Horseradish (2 inch long root)
>
> 1 gallon glass jar

Directions:

Cut the cabbage in quarters and set aside.

Peel and slice the horseradish length wise, in ½ inch slices. They will look lil tick sticks.

On the bottom of the jar, lay thyme and fresh dill.

Add the slices of horseradish (peeled).

Place the cabbage in the glass jar. You can add more slices of horseradish to the sides of the jar.

Prepare the brine: mix salt in filtered water to make a concentrated solution (it should have a strong salty taste).

Pour the brine over the cabbage to cover it. Make sure all the cabbage is submerged.

Leave about a 1 inch of space on top for expansion.

Close the jar with a lid—not too tight to allow the fermentation gasses to escape. Cover the jar with a kitchen towel to keep it in the dark.

Keep it at room temperature to allow it to ferment.

Note: It will take 5-7 days for the sauerkraut juice to be ready.

You can keep the jar on the counter for a very long time. Every time you take out juice, you can replace it with water or brine, and the fermentation process will continue. If you wish to stop it, just transfer the jar to the refrigerator.

You can also consume the cabbage. Just take out one piece, shred it and serve as is or add some olive oil to it.

Enjoy it with meats and eggs. You can add it to the soups as well.

Beetroot Kvass

This is savory probiotic beverage which you can have with your meals to aid stomach acid production and digestion of foods due to its high enzyme and beneficial bacteria content.

Ingredients:

1 medium beetroot

5 cloves of garlic

Ginger root

Horseradish root

Turmeric root

1-2 tbsp. Celtic sea salt (to taste)

2 tbsp. peppercorns

2 tbsp. mustard seeds

1 cup whey or sauerkraut juice, as a starter

Water, filtered or spring

Directions:

Slice the beets finely (do not grate in a food processor, as that will open up the cell walls and release too much sugar, which in turn will make the beet ferment too quickly and produce alcohol).

Peel and slice the garlic.

Cut all the other roots in 1 inch pieces.

Place all the solid ingredients into a 2 liter/quart jar.

Add 1-2 tbsp. Celtic sea salt, 1 cup of whey/sauerkraut juice, and fill the jar with water. Let it ferment in a warm place for 2-5 days. Keep it covered, similarly to the jars of sauerkraut.

After that, keep it in the refrigerator.

Drink it diluted with water. Keep adding water in the jar every time you take out so your kvass will keep going for a long time.

When it starts getting pale, then the beetroot is "consumed," and it is time to make a new batch.

For The Sweet Tooth

Chia Pudding

Makes 1 serving / Net carbs per serving: 8 g

Ingredients:

> 3 tbsp. chia seeds (whole)
>
> 1 cup Pine Nut Hemp Milk (see recipe below, or use any commercial nut milk you prefer)

Directions:

Place the milk in a mason jar.

Add the seeds to the milk.

Close the jar with the lid and shake vigorously for about 30-60 seconds (to prevent the seeds from clumping together).

Place the jar on the counter if you will serve it within an hour, or place it in the refrigerator if you intend to serve it later or the next day.

Note: You can add food grade essential oils to flavor this pudding (lavender, mint, citrus, orange, grapefruit), or use spices like allspice, cardamom, cinnamon, turmeric.

Pine Nut and Hemp Milk

Makes 5 servings / Net carbs per serving: 5.4 g

One serving = 1 cup

Ingredients:

¾ cup pine nuts

½ cup hemp seeds

4 cups water

Pinch of Himalayan salt

1 tbsp. honey

Directions:

Place all the ingredients in a blender (it works best in something like a VitaMix). Blend them for 2 min.

It is ready to serve or to keep in a glass bottle inside the refrigerator of 2-3 days.

Note: You don't need to strain it. However, the solids will separate from the liquid as it sits in the refrigerator. All you need to do is to shake the bottle before you use it. All store bought nut milks use gums to prevent this natural phenomenon of separation. I recommend staying away from gums as much as possible, especially if you are in great need to heal your gut lining.

For more whole foods, low carb-high fat recipes visit:
https://www.mihaelatelecan.com/category/recipes/

FINAL THOUGHTS

In "MAKE PEACE WITH FAT" I tried to address a big piece of our environment that contributes to the health or disease of our very complex body: *food*.

For the vast majority of people, the nutritional protocols described here work and they see results relatively quickly. Please keep in mind that you are not "the majority"; you are a unique individual, and you have your own unique response to food and the environment.

Look at this approach as if it is one of the many Lego® pieces you will need in order to build the Lego® of a "happy, healthy, vibrant life." You will feel an overall improvement in your health and energy. The weight may or may not come off as much or as fast as you may desire. I'm saying this, because I know how much we all want to have that perfect body, to fit in that size of clothing, or to see a certain number on the scale. We want that to happen "yesterday." I agree that the way you look and feel is important, but don't let it be the way you measure your success. The weight loss will eventually follow the rest of the many health outcomes you are going to reap by changing your lifestyle and by following the MRP or the GRP.

Embark on this journey with appreciation and not with expectation; it will be so much easier. Don't expect instant results, as you didn't get sick overnight. Over the course of many years you have been building the Lego® of a "diseased, in pain and frustrated life." Give yourself and your body time to reverse the damage that took place over time.

Last summer, my nephew and I were building a pretty complex Lego®: an antique car. I can't remember exactly how many steps it had, but it had well over 200. It took us three weeks to finally reach the last few steps. We were so excited; the car was looking good. Only when we had to add the wheels did we realize that we did one of the very first steps wrong, something like step 12 or 18. We tried hard to fix it without having to undo the entire Lego®. It was impossible. We had two options: to give up and have a defective car, or to undo the Lego® down to the faulty step, and start rebuilding it, again.

You, at one point in your life, probably built a Lego® too and had to undo it, so you may be able to relate to this. It is actually more difficult and sometimes it takes as long as building it. You need not only time, but the willingness to do that kind work. To take it apart, piece by piece is frustrating, to say the least. You need to have a strong desire to see that final Lego®, built well, in order to do it.

I think building a healthy, happy life is very similar to building a complex Lego® At times we do a few steps wrong or we use the incorrect pieces for the Lego® we are trying to build. We eat the wrong food; we don't move enough, we have too much stress, not enough sleep, etc. The only way to fix it is to be willing to "destroy" the defective Lego® and "rebuild" it sometimes from scratch sometimes more than once. With perseverance it can be done.

There is no quick fix.

Be willing, committed, consistent, and diligent. Trust and appreciate. Cultivate love and joy. Appreciation is key to success. Appreciate and be grateful for the small things in your life that are already working for you. Appreciate even the fact that you had the energy, discipline and the commitment to read this book

Take this journey from a place of self-love. Once a friend of mine said, "You can't heal the body you don't love," and I agree with that.

To heal, you need to love yourself and others around you. You need to believe and trust.

All those emotions are of high vibrating energy. That's the energy of health and healing. When you vibrate high, you make choices that match the vibration state you are in. Think of the healing foods as high frequency foods; they match the emotions of joy, love, happiness, and excitement.

The best way to approach any change is to look at what you are gaining, rather than what you are letting go. Is the cup half full or half empty? They are both correct. What do you choose to see? I hope the half full.

As an example, focus on the abundance and variety of foods you will bring in rather than of those you will let go of.

The first step in health transformation is mindset and belief. As you strengthen the beliefs and power up your mindset for success, you'll begin to take actions and the results will follow.

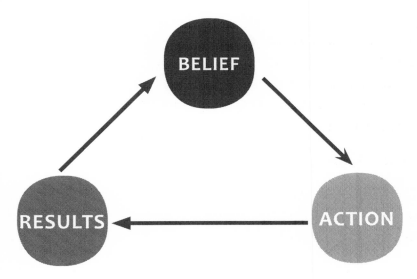

What if you work on your beliefs and you take action, you follow the protocols described here, and you don't get results you've envisioned? What should you do then?

If that's the case, you may want to look at other factors. You need additional Lego® pieces. Keep in mind, you are a very complex "bio-machine." You possess a web of hormones and you have a unique genetic makeup. "How are mine thyroid, adrenal and gonadal (sex) hormone systems functioning? How about genetic variations or mutations, like methylation defects (MTHFR-gene mutation)?"

Trust that you will find all the pieces of the Lego® that will help you build your "healthy, happy, vibrant, life." Begin with the MRP and GRP. If that's not enough to complete your Lego®, investigate further and see what pieces of the Lego® you are missing. You will eventually find them all. Keep building, piece by piece.

Enjoy the journey of health and healing as you aim for your goals, and be ready to go to places you never even dreamed of.

HASSLE FREE HEALING

Mihaela A. Telecan

RECIPES INDEX

NOTES

1.   Angulo Chen, Sandie. "What Did People Eat In The 1800s?" *Ancestry Blog.* 14 Aug. 2017. Web.

2.   Hopkin, Michael. "Ethiopia Is Top Choice for Cradle of Homo Sapiens." *Nature News.* Nature Publishing Group, 16 Feb. 2005. Web.

3.   Sisson, Mark. "What Did Our Ancient Ancestors Actually Eat?" *Mark's Daily Apple.* 17 June 2014. Web.

4.   Weston A. Price. Nutrition and Physical Degeneration, Price- Pottenger Nutrition Foundation, 2012.

.   Gibbons, Ann, and Photographs By Matthieu Paley. "The Evolution of Diet." *National Geographic.* Web.

.   "Insulin." *Merriam-Webster.* Merriam-Webster. Web.

.   "National Center for Health Statistics." *Centers for Disease Control and Prevention.* Centers for Disease Control and Prevention, 03 May 2017. Web.

.   "New CDC Report: More than 100 Million Americans Have Diabetes or Prediabetes." June-July 2017. Web.

.   "Autoimmune Disease Statistics • AARDA." *AARDA.* Web.

.   Fung, Jason, and Jimmy Moore. *The Complete Guide to Fasting: Heal Your Body through Intermittent, Alternate-day, and Extended Fasting.* Victory Belt, 2016. Print.

.   Crofts, C., G. Schofield, C. Zinn, M. Wheldon, and J. Kraft. "Identifying Hyperinsulinaemia in the Absence of Impaired Glucose Tolerance: An Examination of the Kraft Database." *Diabetes Research and Clinical Practice.* U.S. National Library of Medicine, Aug. 2016. Web.

12.   Ridker, Paul M. "High-Sensitivity C-Reactive Protein: Potential Adjunct for Global Risk Assessment in the Primary Prevention of Cardiovascular Disease." *Circulation*. American Heart Association, Inc., 03 Apr. 2001. Web.

13.   "MTHFR Gene - Genetics Home Reference." *U.S. National Library of Medicine*. National Institutes of Health. Web.

14.   Brenner, R. R. "Hormonal Modulation of Delta6 and Delta5 Desaturases: Case of Diabetes." *Prostaglandins, Leukotrienes, and Essential Fatty Acids*. U.S. National Library of Medicine, Feb. 2003. Web.

15.   Nishimura, Satoshi, Ichiro Manabe, and Ryozo Nagai. "Adipose Tissue Inflammation in Obesity and Metabolic Syndrome." *Discovery Medicine*. 22 Sept. 2009. Web.

16.   "Eicosanoid." *Merriam-Webster*. Merriam-Webster. Web.

17.   Crofts, Jeffry Gerber, MD. "Diabetes Is a Vascular Disease – More on Joseph R. Kraft, MD." *Jeffry Gerber, MD - Denver's Diet Doctor*. 20 May 2017. Web. 17 Oct. 2017.

18.   Campbell-McBride, Natasha. *Gut and Psychology Syndrome: Natural Treatment for Autism, Dyspraxia, A.D.D., Dyslexia, A.D.H.D., Depression, Schizophrenia*. Medin form, 2010. Print.

19.   Groff, James L., and Sareen S. Gropper. *Advance of Nutrition and Human Metabolism*. Third ed. Wadsworth, 2000. Print.

20.   Payne, A. N., C. Chassard, and C. Lacroix. "Gut Microbial Adaptation to Dietar Consumption of Fructose, Artificial Sweeteners and Sugar Alcohols: Implication for Host–microbe Interactions Contributing to Obesity." *Obesity Reviews*. Black well Publishing Ltd, 11 June 2012. Web.

21.   Volek, Jeff S., and Stephen D. Phinney. *The Art and Science of Low Carbohydrate Living: An Expert Guide to Making the Life-saving Benefits of Carbohydrate Restriction Sustainable and Enjoyable*. Beyond Obesity, 2011. Print.

22.   Owen, Oliver E. "Ketone Bodies as a Fuel for the Brain during Starvation." Ju 2005. Web.

23.   Greshko, Michael. "How Many Cells Are in the Human Body-And How Ma Microbes?"*National Geographic*. National Geographic Society, 13 Jan. 2016. Web.

24.   Tokunaga, Chiharu, Ken-Ichi Yoshino, and Kazuyoshi Yonezawa. "MTOR tegrates Amino Acid- and Energy-sensing Pathways." *Biochemical and Biophysi*

Research Communications 313.2 (2004): 443-46. Web.

25.   Campbell-McBride, Natasha. *Put Your Heart in Your Mouth!: What Really Is Heart Disease and What Can We Do to Prevent and Even Reverse It.* Medinform, 2012. Print.

26.   Pitchford, Paul. *Healing with Whole Foods: Asian Traditions and Modern Nutrition.* North Atlantic, 2002. Print.

27.   Sugarman, Joe. "Are There Any Proven Benefits to Fasting?" *Johns Hopkins Health Review.* Web.

28.   Mattson, M. P. "Energy Intake, Meal Frequency, and Health: A Neurobiological Perspective." *Annual Review of Nutrition.* U.S. National Library of Medicine, 7 Mar. 20056. Web. 17 Oct. 2017. <https://www.ncbi.nlm.nih.gov/pubmed/16011467>.

29.   Stewart, W. K., and L. W. Fleming. "Features of a Successful Therapeutic Fast of 382 Days' Duration." *Postgraduate Medical Journal* 49.569 (1973): 203-09. Web.

30.   Harris, William S. "The Omega-3 Index as a Risk Factor for Coronary Heart Disease."*The American Journal of Clinical Nutrition.* 01 June 2008. Web.

31.   Center for Food Safety and Applied Nutrition. "Food Additives & Ingredients Overview of Food Ingredients, Additives & Colors." *U S Food and Drug Administration Home Page.* Center for Food Safety and Applied Nutrition, Apr. 2010. Web.

32.   "Pollutants in Fish Inhibit Human's Natural Defense System." *ScienceDaily.* University of California - San Diego, 16 Apr. 2016. Web.

33.   Higdon, Jane. *An Evidence-based Approach to Dietary Phytochemicals.* Thieme, 2007. Print.

34.   Daniel, Kaayla. "Why Broth Is Beautiful: Essential Roles for Proline, Glycine and Gelatin." *The Weston A. Price Foundation.* 18 June 2003. Web.

35.   "Erucic Acid a Possible Health Risk for Highly Exposed Children." *European Food Safety Authority.* 20 Nov. 2016. Web.

36.   "Erucic Acid." *U.S. National Library of Medicine.* National Institutes of Health, Aug. 2008. Web.

37.   "What Are the Guidelines for Percentage of Body Fat Loss?" *ACE Fit | Fitness Information.* 02 Dec. 2009. Web.

38.   Weindruch, R., and RL Walford. "Dietary Restriction in Mice Beginning at

1 Year of Age: Effect on Life-span and Spontaneous Cancer Incidence." *Science.* American Association for the Advancement of Science, 12 Mar. 1982. Web.

39. "Writing S.M.A.R.T. Goals." Web. <http://www.hr.virginia.edu/uploads/documents/media/Writing_SMART_Goals.pdf>.

40. Publishing, Harvard Health. "Glycemic Index and Glycemic Load for 100+ Foods."*Harvard Health.* 27 Aug. 2015. Web.

41. EWG. "EWG's 2017 Shopper's Guide to Pesticides in Produce." *EWG.* Web. 17 Oct. 2017. <https://www.ewg.org/foodnews/dirty_dozen_list.php#.Wb7A3rKGPIU>.

42. Volek, Jeff S., and Stephen D. Phinney. *The Art and Science of Low Carbohydrate Performance.* Beyond Obesity LLC, 2012. Print.

43. Kendall, Marty. "The Blood Glucose, Glucagon and Insulin Response to Protein."*Optimising Nutrition.* 31 July 2017. Web.

44. "How Is Metabolic Syndrome Diagnosed?" *National Heart Lung and Blood Institute.* U.S. Department of Health and Human Services, 22 June 2016. Web.

45. C.Clemente, Jose C., Luke K. Ursell, Laura Wegener Parfrey, and Rob Knight "The Impact of the Gut Microbiota on Human Health: An Integrative View." *Cell* Cell Press, 15 Mar. 2012. Web.

46. "Legume Family." *Dictionary.com.* Dictionary.com, 2017. Web.

47. Jones, David S., MD. *Textbook of Functional Medicine.* Institute for Functiona Medicine, 2005. Print.

48. "NSF Standards." *NSF RSS.* Web.

49. "Diagnosing Diabetes and Learning About Prediabetes." *American Diabete Association.* Web.

50. Mensing, Carolé. *The Art and Science of Diabetes Self-management Educatio A Desk Reference for Healthcare Professionals.* American Association of Diabet Educators, 2006. Print.

51. Mateljan, George. *The World's Healthiest Foods: Essential Guide for the Healt iest Way of Eating.* George Mateljan Foundation, 2007. Print.

52. Mahan, L. Kathleen., and Sylvia Escott-Stump. *Krause's Food, Nutrition, & D Therapy.* Philadelphia: Saunders, 2004. Print.

53. Ali, Norlaily Mohd, Swee Keong Yeap, Wan Yong Ho, Boon Kee Beh, Sheau Wei Tan, and Soon Guan Tan. "The Promising Future of Chia, Salvia HispanicaL." *Journal of Biomedicine and Biotechnology* 2012 (2012): 1-9. Web.

54. Turner, Lori Waite., and Eleanor Noss. Whitney. *Study Guide for Whitney and Rolfes's Understanding Nutrition, Tenth Edition.* Thomson/Wadsworth, 2005. Print.

55. Patricia Burtin, "Nutritional Value of Seaweed." *Electronic Journal of Environmental, Agricultural and Food Chemistry,* ISSN: 1579-4377. Web. <http://docshare01. docshare.tips/files/9389/93899794.pdf>.

56. Katsuki, A., Sumida, Y., Gabazza, E., Murashima, S., Furuta, M., Araki-Sasaki, R., Hori, Y., Yano, Y. and Adachi, Y. (2018). *Homeostasis Model Assessment Is a Reliable Indicator of Insulin Resistance During Follow-up of Patients With Type 2 Diabetes.* [online] Available at: http://care.diabetesjournals.org/content/24/2/362 [Accessed 12 Sep. 2018].

INDEX

Made in the USA
Middletown, DE
10 November 2018